End Self-Sabotage and Stop Fighting with Yourself

Uncover and Overcome Root Causes of Addictive Self-Destructive Behavior through Self-Awareness, Self-Belief and an Empowered Positive Mindset

Jackson James

3 eye publishing

The +Point. The Power of Positive Thinking for Everyone!

Jackson James

End Self-Sabotage and Stop Fighting with Yourself!

Book Cover by Olina

1st edition 2024

Jackson James, Author of The +Point; The Power of Positive Thinking for Everyone!

Contents

A Big Hello from Ring Side

"We sabotage the great things in our lives because deep down, we don't feel worthy of having great things." [1]

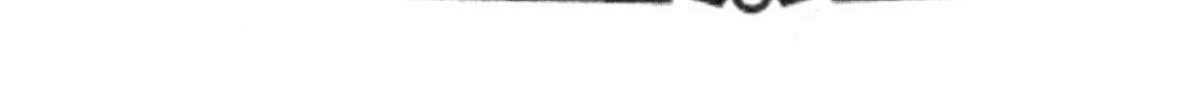

Seconds Out, Round One!

Hello Everyone!

I'm Jackson James, and I will be your guide, if you will have me, on this amazing journey to unearth the transformative power that lurks within each of us. Buckle up, because we're about to embark on an extraordinary adventure – a quest to unravel the mysteries of self-sabotage and dis-

---

1.

cover the miraculous cure for those destructive tendencies of ours. Together we will genuinely make a truly gigantum leap into the uncharted realms of your greater more positive self to release the full potential that awaits just beneath the surface. In short, I will show you how to stop fighting yourself and start to live a successful, fulfilled, and happy life.

So who is Jackson James anyway?

A great question and one which is inevitably and often followed by "How can this guy help me?". Well, let me spill the beans. Born and bred in the bustling heart of London, England, I've navigated through life's twists and turns, sipping lattes and enjoying the vibrancy of red buses that go too slow and black taxis that generally hurtle around like Hotwheel pace cars. I was educated in the illustrious halls of Cambridge, much to my old man's delight, and then I took a detour from the conventional path, exploring the world instead of diving into a typical nine-to-five gig. Much to my old man's dislike.

My journeys have taken me across Europe, Asia, and of course, the States, where I have worked with the corporate big boys (and big girls), shaping businesses and their employee interactions, whilst using my masterly education in Psychology and Positive Psychology to ever greater effect. Oh, and I have also written the odd book on the subject. For now, I split my time between the Bay Area of San Francisco and London where I grew up. During all this time, referred to as 'The wasted years' by pops, I have studied the innate human ability to interact with others, influence, cajole, or generally intimidate to generate the outcomes either they wanted or didn't want to happen. Yes, human interaction either at work, at home, or just down the pub can be a tricky and fascinating thing all at the same time. During my many years of research, I have discovered an awful lot about human behavior and its effects on others and themselves. Many a negative outcome has been reached by otherwise successful people who at times find themselves hell-bent on self-sabotage. This happens as much in our personal lives as it does in our business lives and can lead to a downward spiral of negative behavior that limits our potential to succeed. Worst of all this type of behavior can become habit-forming leading to repeated bouts of self-destruction with their associated impacts on our daily lives. If this is something that begins to resonate with you, then this book will certainly be for you. For those of you who can't recognize these sometimes subtle tell-tell signs then let me just say that recognition and understanding are the first keys to unlocking the menace that is self-sabotage, and we will be covering that too. So basically what I'm saying is that this book will be a boon to all of you irrespective of whatever stage of your life, career, or relationship you are at, whether you are male, female, or indeed any other assigned gender preference.

What are this Book's Objectives?

Well, you could also ask what is all this fuss about self-sabotage anyway? Surely we can skip the whole book-buying and reading thing and just get on with our lives and see what happens? Well, my friends, the world is brimming with amazing opportunities, yet we often find ourselves entangled in the web of our own undoing. Being tripped up in our pursuits of happiness is one thing but it's far worse if you are the one doing the tripping. So this book is designed to tackle the issue using proven methods that recognize, address, and provide repeatable solutions as a means to counteract self-sabotaging tendencies bringing positivity, motivation, and success into your life. This book also isn't your run-of-the-mill self-help spiel, regurgitated time and again to grab book sales and make a living out of acquiring members for paid-for self-help groups. It's a call to arms, a journey of self-discovery, and a blueprint for those seeking to break free from the chains of self-sabotage, personal destruction, and debilitating negativity.

As we dive into the pages that follow, you'll encounter a unique blend of wisdom, exercises, and knowledge drizzled with a splash of humor, all designed to flip your internal switch from negativity to positivity. But here's the kicker – it's not just about business or personal life. This book defies the norms; it's for everyone, young or old, alive or dead. You can wield these strategies at any juncture of life, or afterlife, reshaping your existence, or non-existence, in the most positive ways imaginable. And it's all contained here in one awesome tome of knowledge gently held within a slick shiny cover unless you cheaped out and got a download instead.. where you will of course be saving trees.

There's just one other thing to mention before we get started. I am a lover of good grammar. I do respect it and a book with correct punctuation and grammar is a joy to read. This is not one of those books. Sorry for you competing grammar lovers out there. I have ignored some, well a lot, of the stricture and structure that come with writing a correctly edited and well-grammared book simply because we are going to have a conversation and I simply don't talk like that. I tend to start sentences with And or Because for instance and a whole load of Buts. I did try to follow the rules but I really don't think that you will likely talk that way either, so for all grammar aficionados, please don't judge me.

The Importance of Self-Discovery.

Now, let's jump forward and talk about your brain – a colossal powerhouse with 86 billion neurons, zapping information quicker than a speeding helicopter, and capable of producing enough electricity to light a decent-sized lightbulb. Impressive, right? Yet, we often let this magnificent organ dwell in the dark realms of negativity, fixating on trivial issues like lukewarm lattes or untamed grass verges. Imagine a world where your brilliant brain was set free to unleash its computable genius upon the world in search of success without someone, possibly yourself, hitting the delete button. Imagine all those countless occasions when you reset factory settings rather than pursue the world of opportunities that existed for you because something held you back and it was determined to sabotage your success! That is what I'm talking about when I refer to self-discovery. It is a means of unchaining yourself from the restrictions that you place by establishing the root causes and the reasons why you can be self-destructive.

The journey we're about to undertake isn't just about positive thinking; it's a call to explore the untapped potential that lies within us all. It's about making decisions that defy adversity, creating a world where positivity, motivation, and self-belief reign supreme and our tendencies to sabotage ourselves are both understood and overcome. Imagine a life where minor hiccups don't ruffle your feathers, and your energy is channeled into the positive aspects of your life, be that your career or the deepening of your relationships. These are the realms that we're aiming for and these are the opportunities that lie ahead.

Let me share a secret. This isn't a book of reinterpreted age-old ideas. What lies ahead of you is a fusion of innovative exercises and knowledge transfer, a powerful concoction that has already been proven to work wonders in my life and the lives of the many whom I have worked with. This isn't just a journey; it's an invitation to establish a life teeming with optimism, resilience, and infinite possibilities built on self-belief, positive approaches, and inspiring results. Join now the many who have traversed this path of enlightenment starting with self-exploration and discovery and ending with a resilient life built to grasp every opportunity that life gives without constantly f*cking it all up.

As we stride through each chapter, I'll provide insights and examples to help you gain a full awareness of the issues surrounding self-sabotage and offer simple step-by-step solutions to overcome them. I will act as your guide, mentor, and ringmaster, navigating the twists and turns of self-discovery and personal development. We will follow along a proven path of transformation where we will gain awareness, embrace our acceptance, adopt new approaches, and finally advocate the results of our quest. This linear process will guide you along the road of resilience and fortitude until you reach the destination of strength and self-belief. Together, we'll rewrite the script of your life, illuminating that route to ongoing success in all that you do. Brace yourself – this journey will change your thinking and levels of understanding so that you can make the critical changes needed to end self-sabotage.

The bell is ringing – let's grab the ropes and with a flourish spring purposefully into the ring ready to take on our self-sabotaging demons and uncover the magic and success that lies within!

Chapter One

Recognizing Subtle Self-Sabotage Cues

"Sometimes we are our own worst enemy, and the biggest obstacle to achieving our goals is the doubt we harbor within ourselves." [1]

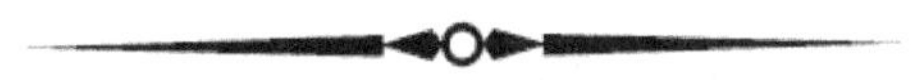

Hello and welcome on this expedition of self-discovery. In this chapter, we will unravel the intricate nature of self-sabotage. As we set sail into this uncharted territory, our compass is pointed toward understanding and awareness of the subtle cues that often go unnoticed but wield tremendous influence over our lives. Buckle up, for the journey promises to be both eye-opening and transformative.

Let's go!

1.

Awareness and Understanding Make for Good Bed-Fellows

If you wish to get to grips with something that you would like to change then you must first gain an awareness and understanding of exactly what that something is and how it is affecting you. This makes logical sense right? However, when it comes to ourselves and our behavior it is not always easy to spot the wood for the trees even if you may possess a mighty big chainsaw. That's because we are highly adaptable creatures. We quickly adapt to situations around us and change our viewpoint accordingly even if we don't tell ourselves that we are doing it. We can apply that logic to relationships. We may start a relationship full of enthusiasm, excitement, and vigor ensuring that we do everything in our power to satisfy the focus of our attention but a year or two later things often change. What was new and exciting may have become accepted and routine. The effort that we give the relationship may have waned as our priorities outshine the priorities of our partner. We often look back and wonder why a relationship stagnates and fails blaming the other for the situation. Now this example can be applied to multiple scenarios all owing their failings to a lack of self-awareness and understanding of the situation unfolding around us and a lack of care and attention.

In many situations, we need to first examine ourselves and avoid blaming others for our misfortunes. This has never been more truer than when addressing self-sabotaging tendencies. We often look outward rather than inward tending to blame the situation or the circumstance, other people, or even the weather. As human beings, we are used to habitually passing the buck. This blame dodging allows us to feel just a little bit better about the situation and at the same time avoids all that head-scratching spent on understanding. But whilst it may alleviate our feelings of being fully or even partly responsible it doesn't help us to deal with the reason why and without dealing with that simple three-letter word we are just going to keep repeating the same behaviors over and over again.

This brings us fairly neatly back to where we started; gaining awareness and understanding of our self-sabotaging tendencies. Once we ask ourselves the 'Why' question when situations repeat or even before, we can start down the road to self-discovery and recovery. Now for this, you are already off to a flying start because you have decided to read this book. You have chosen the topic, selected the book (thank you), and have gotten through the quirky introduction and are still reading. Something inside of you has already jumped up, waved its arms wildly about, and shouted loud enough to be overheard above the background noise of life. It's telling you that you need to invest time in understanding the full impact that self-destructive tendencies are inflicting on your life and those around you.

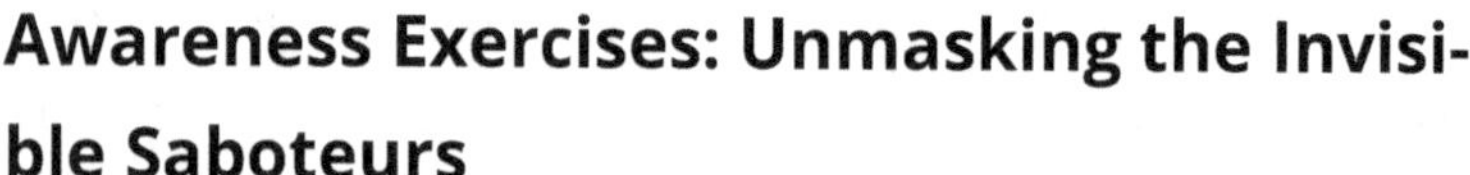

Awareness Exercises: Unmasking the Invisible Saboteurs

I know that it's only Chapter One and I am already lining up some tasks for you to undertake. It's early but I already have faith in your determination to succeed.

With any transformation, personal or business, human or technological, we need to start with awareness. I recently worked with a well-known furniture retailer to re-examine how they delivered on their global marketing and customer relationships. To effectively achieve the changes necessary to keep that business performing well we needed to first create broad awareness. This awareness covered existing working practices and the future desired state with all the waypoints in between. It spanned the world involving culturally diverse teams across multiple functions and responsibilities. This awareness once delivered created a globally 'common' foundation of understanding on which to build the requisite changes necessary for improvement. It also highlighted the reason 'Why' - without change to a common approach they would slowly lead the business to extinction. Now apply that business logic to your own needs. Why do you need to change? What are the signs that scream out to you? What made you search out and select this book in the first place? Let's take a moment to explore deep inside your grey matter to discover the answers:

Each of the following exercises requires a quiet space to conduct. So before starting, grab yourself a comfy chair and some quiet alone time. Try to ensure that you conduct all of the exercises from this book in a place that you feel both physically and emotionally comfortable in. A journal, a big one, is also a vital requirement as you will use it to capture your thoughts for later reflection.

1. The Procrastination Puzzle: The Art of Delay

(15 minutes)

Procrastination, the silent saboteur, is an affliction that often creeps into our lives unnoticed. It's not just about delaying tasks; it's about the underlying motives and the psychological dance we engage in with ourselves when action or decision-making is required. Do you suffer from procrastination? If so complete the following exercise and consider all the moments when you pushed things to the last minute and the palpable stress that ensued because of it.

- **Reflection:** Dive deep into the reasons behind your procrastination. Is it a coping mechanism driven by a fear of failure, or a rebellion against imposed timelines? Spend at least five minutes considering the question before completing the exercise. Be completely honest and open with yourself to gain the full benefits of all of the exercises. Gaining an understanding of the causes of your procrastination will be crucial.

- **Personal Exploration:** Now I would like you to recall a specific instance of procrastination. Concentrate on that and try to remember and re-feel the emotions that surfaced. Try to discover what deeper motivations were at play. Understanding the emotional landscape will provide you with valuable insights that we will use later on.

2. Overcommitment Overload: The Juggling Act Gone Wrong

(15 minutes)

Did you know that the constant need to say "yes" can be a guise for self-sabotage? Overcommitting often leads to burnout, affecting not only the quality of our work but also our mental and emotional well-being. Overcommitment can extend to loved ones, family and friends, and even less well-known acquaintances. If you know that you overcommit then complete the exercises below.

- **Reflection:** Take a moment to examine instances where overcommitment has led to an overwhelming sense of stress. What compelled you to take on more than you could handle and did you instinctively know this at the time of agreeing to it?

Thinking back can you remember and capture the emotions that drove your behavior?

- **Setting Personal Boundaries:** Reflect on the importance of setting healthy boundaries. When and where do you struggle to say "no," and what fears arise in asserting your limits? Do these fears link to any other difficulties you have experienced? Capture these all down in a journal for later review.

3. The Comfort Zone Conundrum: Where Growth Stagnates

(15 minutes)

For those who don't recognize the term 'Comfort Zone,' it is when actions or decision-making regarding a certain topic feel easy to undertake because they deal with known quantities or situations that you have comfortably experienced in the past. The comfort zone, while as the name suggests is comforting, can also become a breeding ground for self-sabotage and self-limiting beliefs in your advancement. Recognizing when you resist stepping outside this zone is pivotal for personal growth.

- **Reflection:** For this exercise explore situations where the allure of the familiar has held you back from trying something new. What fears or limiting beliefs kept you in the confines of what you already knew?

- **Exploration Challenge:** Identify one area in your life where you are currently resisting change. Does this resistance stem from not wishing to step outside of your comfort zone? What small steps can you take to challenge this resistance and invite growth? What are the perils that exist if you do this?

4. Anger Management: The Emotional Furnace

(15 minutes)

Do certain situations get you all fired up inside? Do you feel your anger rising as you get stressed or anxious? Do you experience the flight or fight emotional tug or war far more often than you would like and does it lead to rash decision-making and potentially destructive actions? All these described situations indicate a need to manage the anger bubbling away just beneath the surface.

- **Reflection:** Take a quiet moment to consider the last bout of anger that you experienced. Was it premeditated or did it take you by surprise, rising from your inner depths like a piping hot geezer? Outside of the anger itself, what other emotions did you experience immediately preceding and after?

- **Pattern Exploration**: Have you experienced those same emotions before in a similar situation? If so spend a few moments exploring the feelings that flowed with it. Were they the same? Now consider what was driving those feelings and if they occur in any similar situations where your anger swells. What connects the situations and what patterns are materializing?

Remember to take your time and explore in detail the questions posed. Their purpose is to establish a foothold for the inquisitive practice of self-reflection. To think beneath the perceived need and establish an awareness not only of the impact that self-sabotage may be having in your life but also to start to highlight emotional drivers.

Guided Reflections: Journey into Your Inner Cosmos

I hope that you were able to explore your emotions to answer the previous questions. If you find it difficult, don't worry. This is a new skill that we are developing and it will take time, and further exercises, to hone into shape. Self-reflection is a valuable technique to learn as it forms the basis of a transferable skill, one which aids broader understanding and problem-solving. We will now develop this to the next stage by exploring some journaling exercises.

1. Self-Sabotage Journaling: Pattern Recognition

(2 weeks)

Over the next fourteen days, your journal will become a constant companion and compass, guiding you through the labyrinth of your self-sabotaging tendencies. If you have not done so already it's time to invest in a journal to capture your progress. Once you have one I want you to use it to record instances, thoughts, and emotions, that you experience throughout our time together. These changes to your emotional state could occur anywhere, at work, at home, or even when you socialize. Ideally, use the journal at all times. As you notice a change in your emotional state linked to instances where self-sabotaging occurs note them down. Examples could include instances when you feel constrained to remain in your comfort zone or feel threatened by change. It could exhibit itself in bouts of anger or frustration or through a lack of patience when met by certain situations that threaten your sense of order or control. By faithfully recording these occurrences you will be creating a roadmap to your behavioral patterns. This will become invaluable as we explore deeper into your psyche.

Include the following:

- **Insightful Inquiry:** Review your journal daily for recurring themes. What patterns emerge, and are there specific triggers that consistently lead to self-sabotaging feelings or actions? Highlight those reoccurring instances and note the specific triggers involved.

- **Pattern Recognition:** Examine your journal entries for those highlighted commonalities. Are there specific situations or emotional states that precede your self-sabotaging behaviors? This may be a hard thing to recognize but believe me when I say that this will become the key to unlocking self-sabotage controls. Don't worry if you can't recall and capture all these instances as we will explore this topic in far greater detail later.

2. Timeline of Choices: Deciphering Crossroads

(45 minutes)

Our life is a tapestry woven with the choices that we make. Should I get up? What cereal should I eat? and Should I try the out-of-date milk? However, some choices hold far greater significance than others and can have a shaping effect on our lives. These could be broad and varied from deciding whether to go for that job promotion to deciding how to proceed with a personal relationship. These decisions we will now explore. For the following exercise, you will require either an A4 journal page or a separate sheet, some coloring pens or pencils, and a yellow highlighter.

First I want you to create a timeline of the most significant decisions that you have made in your life so far. These could be, which college to attend, which boy or girl to date, which job to go for, or which friend to rely on. These critical decisions should cover both personal and work-related situations. Write down each key decision made and the real reason behind why you made them. Draw a simple timeline capturing them down in the order you made them. Scrutinize each decision. What were the emotional drivers that led to it? Was it a good or bad decision and above all was self-sabotage involved in the decision-making process? Run the timelines alongside each other in parallel. A black line should be used leading up to the decision and then a green, red, or blue line should follow. Use green if the decision reached held a positive outcome, red if it was a negative outcome, and blue if it was neither good nor bad. Extend the line if it directly leads to another critical decision point and do the same again. Use your work of art to address the following exercises.

- **Introspective Inquiry:** Reflect on the outcomes of your pivotal life choices. Specifically, focus on the ones that were influenced by your self-sabotage tendencies. How did self-sabotage manifest itself, and what alternative paths could have been taken? Ask yourself if the result would have been different if a different path had been chosen and estimate the level of impact that the choice had upon your life.

- **Decision Awareness:** As you go through the following two weeks take time to consider the significant decisions that you are currently making and why you are making them. Pause and reflect; are there echoes of past self-sabotaging choices influencing your current mindset?

3. Emotional Checkpoint: Navigating Your Inner Weather

(15 minutes)

Emotions provide direction in the tumultuous sea of decision-making. Over the next few weeks, I want you to check in regularly with your emotional state, especially during crucial decision-making junctures. This will be important to establish the level of impact self-sabotaging decision-making is still having on your life and to what degree this changes as you continue to progress through this book.

- **Inner Exploration:** Dive into the emotions accompanying critical decisions. Are there patterns of fear, self-doubt, or unworthiness? How do these emotions influence your choices? If not what other emotions are present and how do these impact?

- **Decision-Making Insights:** Before making a decision, acknowledge and name the emotions present. Capture these down in your journal along with the decision made and later determine if it was a correct decision. Ask yourself how might recognizing and understanding these emotions impact the choices that you make.

These exercises are designed to establish a level of awareness of the impact that self-sabotage has and is having on your life. You may have chosen to explore this area because you already instinctively knew that you were being negatively affected by your tendencies or perhaps this has been a deep awakening of your self-awareness. Either way, it is important to establish an honest baseline of understanding establishing the true impact of self-sabotage upon your life. Gaining such self-awareness builds a firm foundation on which to build supportive solutions that enable you to regain control of your life.

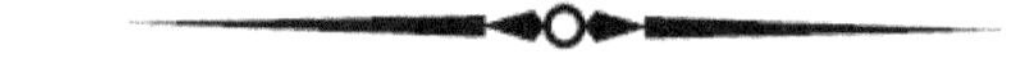

The Broader Impact of Self-Sabotage: Decoding Life's Landscape

I can already see that you are motoring along the expressway of recognition. Know that any sense of darkness encroaching upon your life through self-destructive tendencies, will be vanquished by the light and hope that lies ahead. Our lives are super exciting because they are filled with incredible opportunities. Opportunities to grow, learn, to transform, and to succeed. Just because when we look back the past holds some undesirable aspects to it, doesn't mean that the future has to follow the same path.

You are the owner of your destiny and only you can decide which course it should take from now on. You can decide to navigate to a sunnier clime or choose an extended stay in

Luton. We all have the power to change our futures. Many may sit in fear of that change but it exists all the same like Marmite and cheese on toast – don't knock it until you try it. We will come to change strategies a little later but for now, let us concentrate on nailing the topic of understanding once and for all

Until now you may have thought that self-sabotage only happens to you. This is not at all the case. Take some comfort in the fact that millions of people suffer the exact same affliction, day in, and day out. As you are reading this chapter, literally millions of decisions are being made under the mantel of fear and self-loathing. These decisions are highly likely to negatively impact many of those who are making them as well as those affected by them. Just take a look at today's news headlines, if you dare, for a glimpse of the catastrophic decisions that are being made, many of which will be destructive for the decision-makers as well as those directly and indirectly impacted. Scary isn't it...With that in mind, I would like to introduce the next exercise to you– The Ripple Effect.

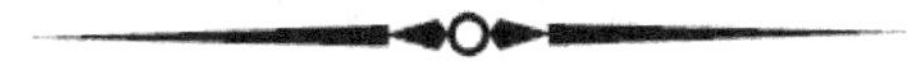

1. The Ripple Effect: A Stone in Life's Pond

(15 minutes)

Like ripples in a pond, self-sabotage extends its influence beyond the immediate. It negatively affects relationships, career trajectories, and overall well-being. Take a few quiet moments to conduct the next exercises to establish further awareness of this effect.

- **Reflective Inquiry:** If you completed the timeline exercise then this would be a good time to pull out your artwork and examine some of what it indicates. Follow your drawn timelines to critical life decision junctures impacted by self-sabotage tendencies. Do any of them intersect or lead to further decisions? What impacts have you noted down from them? Contemplate how self-sabotage in one area might permeate into others. What interconnected patterns can you discern, and how have they shaped your life?

- **Interconnected Choices:** Explore how choices influenced by self-sabotage in one aspect of life may echo or influence other realms. How can breaking these patterns impact your overall journey? For better or for poorer? Note down your findings in your journal, using a separate page and heading it -"**How my self-sabotage thinking has impacted my life**". It may feel harsh, I know it does, but facing your fears and understanding your enemy is the first stage to defeating it.

2. The Slow Erosion: When Drops Become a Deluge

(15 minutes)

Subtle self-sabotage isn't a raging tempest; it's the slow erosion of your potential. Each seemingly insignificant choice contributes to the overall impact on our lives and to those around us.

- **Contemplative Inquiry:** Contemplate the long-term impact of subtle self-sabotage on your goals. How have your negatively influenced decisions shaped your journey until now? Once you have considered these then ask yourself what alternate paths could have been taken. What greater potential could you have realized?

- **Vision for Change:** Now envision a life completely free from the erosion of self-sabotage, where each decision is made in your best interest and that of those around you. What possibilities could unfold when each one of your choices aligns with your true potential? What levels of success could you attain? Where would your career be if you had made more positive decisions? How would your relationships have faired? What about your health and well-being?

Now take your thoughts and answers from these last two exercises and write them down on a new page in your journal and head it – **"This is my true potential"**

3. Breaking the Chains: A Journey to Liberation

(15 minutes)

Recognizing the subtlety of self-sabotage to shape your life is the first step toward breaking free from its tenacious grip. Understanding its real impact on your life and on those around you empowers you to reclaim control over your narrative. Believe me, before you believe yourself in this regard, the opportunity for change always exists irrespective of your past or your present situation. You hold the power to maximize your potential.

Now try these two quick exercises:

- **Empowering Inquiry:** Envision your life unbound by the subtle chains of self-sabotage. How would your journey from today onward unfold if you could navigate without these unseen obstacles? What would you determine to do differently?

- **Liberating Choices:** Now identify just one small but important change that you can make today, I mean right now, to disrupt your pattern of self-sabotaging. What would it be? What liberating choices can you embrace to rewrite the script of your life to come?

Take your responses from these last two questions and write them down on another clean page in your journal. Title that page – **"The changes I will make for success"**

—◦—

Conclusion: Illuminating the Shadows

Wow! I know I have hit you hard in the first chapter with several quick-fire exercises. It is essential early on to establish your reasons to keep reading, learning, and moving forward. If you have reached this point and don't feel motivated or driven by what you have just read then I recommend that you go no further. If you are reading this as part of the free Kindle book sample then close it and look elsewhere. You may not be ready for change right now but also know that that is OK. When you are you can come back and we can try again.

For those of you who bask in the newfound awareness blooming within then welcome to the next stage of your life. We have not merely scratched the surface; we've already delved deep into the recesses of self-sabotage to discover self-awareness and understanding which will form the bedrock of your motivation for change. The journey ahead holds the promise of transformation as we unravel the unconscious patterns that underlie these subtle self-sabotaging cues. So, until we reconvene in the next chapter, let the flame of curiosity burn bright, let introspection be your guide, and may the light of awareness pave your path toward self-discovery.

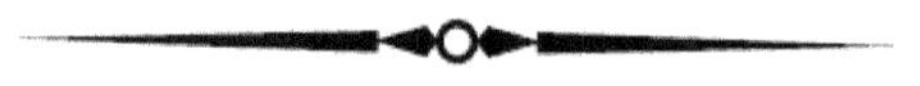

Chapter Two

Exploring the Unconscious

"Self-sabotage is like a game of mental tug-of-war. It is the conscious mind versus the subconscious mind where the subconscious mind always eventually wins." [1]

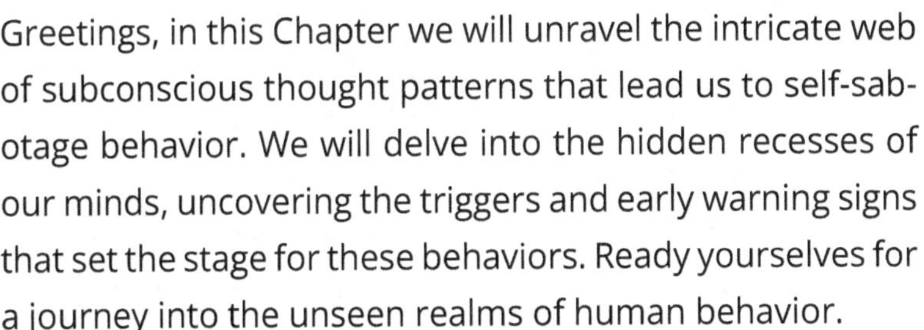

Greetings, in this Chapter we will unravel the intricate web of subconscious thought patterns that lead us to self-sabotage behavior. We will delve into the hidden recesses of our minds, uncovering the triggers and early warning signs that set the stage for these behaviors. Ready yourselves for a journey into the unseen realms of human behavior.

---

1. Bi Bennett,(n.d.), 2024, End Self-Sabotage and Stop Fighting with Yourself!

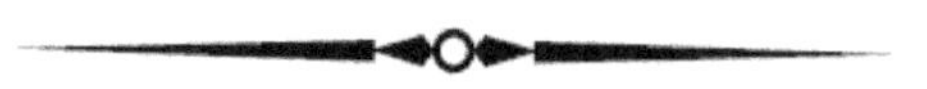

Brain Hacking

Our brains are super complicated and capable of achieving amazing things such as understanding tax returns and knowing the off-side rule. The brain is so amazing that we don't even need to be thinking about something for it to be actively doing that something all on our behalf. This is known as our subconscious which is not too dissimilar to an unregulated Google search engine. There we are all snuggled up and asleep at our office desk whilst our subconscious is whirring away, filling in for us and thinking about the next great thing. It also employs this act of self-will when we are wide awake and still sitting at that same desk answering questions and making decisions. It is here where the problems really start. We inevitably believe that we are in full control of what our brain is doing. We may give it some latitude to do its own thing whilst we are sleep granted, but once we open our bleary eyes to peer out from beneath the duvet we assume that we instantly take back full control. I mean how else could we select the right toothbrush in the morning or match our socks? This is a fundamental error of judgment on our part, for as I have just mentioned our subconscious is still working away doing its own thing affecting everything we thought we were in control of. Just think for instance of how many times you have looked down and found that you are wearing unmatching socks!

Now the point here is that your subconscious acts to steer your behavior based on many things, most of which are too tricky to explain without boring those socks right off your feet. Needless to say, those of us suffering from a bout of self-sabotage will find it lurking somewhere within our subconsciousness, waiting for its moment to strike. This could happen at any time, at home, at work, with friends, or even with loved ones. The important thing to understand is that there is always a precursor to its arrival. A 'tell' that lets you know that something is about to happen. This normally exists as a certain feeling or emotion. You may have felt it. A rising sensation of anxiousness or frustration, of anger or fear. This is the moment that your subconscious pops its head up and signals its imminent arrival and that it's about to influence you. This is the moment just before your self-sabotaging tendencies kick your legs out from under you. Just think of how powerful it would be if you could not only detect that precursor but also do something to counteract your subconscious all before any destructive notion has been acted upon. Neat eh?

So with that in mind let's explore some interesting exercises to do just that.

Uncovering Hidden Patterns and Triggers

1. The Subtle Art of Self-Observation

Self-observation will help us navigate the intricate landscape of our unconscious thought patterns. Through exercises and mindful practices, we will unveil the covert triggers that set off our self-sabotage tendencies.

- **Trigger Identification:** This task links directly with the Self-Sabotage Journaling exercise from Chapter 1. In it, you have spent time capturing all of the incidents where Self-Sabotage negatively encroaches upon your behavior and decision-making. Now I would like you to take that introspective one stage further by identifying the triggers that prompted the emotional shifts and each bout of destructive behavior. As you examine each instance note down the trigger that prompted it.

- **Mindful Exploration:** During the same two weeks I ask you to engage in daily moments of self-observation. This will require a calm environment without disturbances or interruption, so choose your moments well. I would recommend thirty minutes before going to bed. Once you have fully relaxed I want you to review that day's journal entries. Consider which thoughts preceded your self-sabotaging behaviors, and are there recurring themes? Perhaps you feel the blood rushing to your head, or a tendency to switch off from conversations? Maybe you are affected by a strong desire to walk away or to leave the conversation or even an overwhelming upsurge of intense anger. Take the time each day to reflect and uncover these secret signals and check to see if they are symptomatic of further instances of destructive decision-making that you have experienced in the past.

2. The Tapestry of Triggers: Thread by Thread

Following on from the first exercises I want you to concentrate on the triggers that spark those self-sabotage feelings. Triggers act as the threads weaving the tapestry of self-sabotage stimulation. By examining these triggers, you will gain insights into the intricate patterns governing your behaviors.

- **Trigger Mapping:** This exercise is similar to the Timeline of Choices exercise in Chapter One. After two weeks of self-observation and journalling use the same resources to create your personal trigger map. This is like a treasure map identifying the interconnectedness of our self-sabotage feelings. First, write down on the sheet of paper each of the self-sabotage occurrences that have happened during your period of observation. If you have not had too many of those over that period then use previous occurrences. Once you have them all noted draw any lines of intersection noting similar situations or triggers as you go. Color in red any situations that consistently lead to self-sabotage and use green for those which on reflection were not self-sabotage and led to positive outcomes. What threads connect these triggers, and what overarching patterns emerge?

- **Pattern Recognition:** Identify commonalities in the triggers for situations across different aspects of life. How do patterns manifest themselves in relationships, at work, and during personal endeavors? Note these down in your journal under the title **"My Trigger Patterns".**

- **Emotional Check-in:** Now for the most important exercise of all. Linking in with **The Mindful Exploration** above I would like you to examine each of the feelings or sensations that you felt immediately before self-sabotage. Run through each occurrence one by one ensuring each has a list of the emotions that you felt just prior. Once you have them all down written next to each episode I want you to carefully examine your map. What stands out? Are there similar triggers to similar situations and if so are they preempted by the same set of emotions? Do you recognize them and can recall how they affected you at the time? Try to relive them and understand them, drawing no conclusion but merely recognizing them along with their intensity. Grab another clean page and write a heading that reads, **"Self-Sabotage Summary Map "**. Create four columns headed **'Situation, Trigger, Feelings, and Self-Sabotage'.** and list the situation, the trigger, the preceding feelings, and the self-destructive response. Do this for each situation. It could go something like this:

Situation: Leading meeting at work

Trigger: Criticism when providing direction

Feelings: Flushed face, hot and uncomfortable and angry

Self-Sabotage: Expressing agitation and anger, shouting, closing conversations down, and ending the meeting early

Once you have completed these tasks you are well on your way to identifying the emotions that preceded the numerous situations that led to instances of self-sabotage. You now have a full list of occurrences and have identified which ones are destructive, where they occurred the trigger, and the emotions leading to them. Now let's augment that depth of understanding within a new environment. One where your eyes are closed and your subconscious is truly free to wander off and get lost.

The Uncharted Realms of Dreams

Why Do We Dream?

Dreams, often shrouded in mystery, serve as the mind's nocturnal playground where our subconscious takes the spotlight whilst our conscious is taking a much-needed break. While the exact purpose of dreaming remains a subject of significant scientific debate, several theories attempt to unravel this enigma.

Evolutionary Perspective:

From an evolutionary standpoint, some scientists propose that dreaming serves as a mechanism for threat simulation. Something like, "What's that coming over the hill? Oh... it's a monster, a monster!" By simulating challenging scenarios during periods of sleep, our ancestors might have enhanced their ability to handle real-life challenges and not get eaten.

Neurobiological Explanations:

Scientifically, dreaming is closely tied to our sleep cycle, particularly the rapid eye movement (REM) stage. During REM, normally ninety or more minutes into a good night's sleep, the brain activity resembles that of our waking hours, with heightened neural firing and vivid imagery. This phase is integral to memory consolidation and emotional regulation.

Psychological Theories:

One of the more prevalent perspectives suggests that

dreams play a role in processing our emotions, memories, and experiences. They act as a mental rehearsal space, allowing the brain to examine, consolidate information, solve problems, and navigate emotional landscapes.

In essence, while the exact purpose of dreaming remains undetermined, dreams are woven into the fabric of our psychological and neurobiological landscapes, offering a captivating realm for exploration and interpretation and one that can shape how we interpret and respond to situations that we find ourselves in. Our dreams are like a freestyle dance-off, choreographed by the intertwining forces of memory, emotion, and our subconscious. They offer a gateway to the untouched realms of our thoughts, fears, and desires.

The Language of Dreams: How Do We Dream?

Picture your mind as a grand theater, where dreams unfold in acts and scenes. As we sleep, our brain weaves intricate narratives, painting vivid images on the canvas of our imagination. Dreams come in various forms – fleeting fragments, epic sagas, or surreal landscapes. Night after night, we are cast as the lead in a play directed by the mysterious conductor of our subconscious.

Interpreting dreams is therefore a bit like deciphering an ancient manuscript. Symbols, metaphors, and emotions intertwine, creating a rich and powerful tapestry of meaning. Through our dreams, we are conversing with the deepest layers of our being, exploring dimensions inaccessible to us during our waking hours.

Decoding the Dreamscape: What Do Our Dreams Reveal?

So, we have determined that dreams are 'pretty cool' and represent the unfiltered glimpses into our inner world. They spotlight buried thoughts, fears, and unresolved issues, often nudging us to pay close attention to aspects that we may otherwise overlook or back away from during the hustle and bustle of our waking lives. For those of us grappling with self-sabotage tendencies, dreams become a mirror reflecting the subconscious struggles that battle it out inside of us. Unraveling their symbolism can therefore offer us valuable insights into the root causes of our self-destructive behaviors. Now you can see where I'm going with all this dream stuff... Let's explore a bit further.

Facing the Shadows: Confronting Our Self-Sabotage in Our Dreams

Ever find yourself plummeting from great heights or navigating intricate and never-ending mazes in your dreams? These scenarios may hold the key to understanding our self-sabotage tendencies. Dreams often vividly manifest our deepest anxieties and unresolved conflicts. Think of the times when you have been under a lot of stress about a situation and find that it stalks you in your dreams. Acknowledging these dreams provides us with a fantastic opportunity for self-reflection. They are our backstage pass to our psyche's rehearsal, where we can confront fears and in doing so rewrite the script. With skill, we can repeatedly turn our dream world into a therapeutic space for a transformative journey to help end our self-sabotaging tendencies.

Lucid Dreaming: A Step-by-Step Guide to Self-Empowerment

So imagine the opportunity for self-awareness and understanding that using your dreams could present. Think of just how useful it would be to shape your dreams to act as your very own repeat, delete, and rescript buttons for your life, where you could review your choices and select the one with the best outcome to take forward. It's like multivariable testing all taking place within your subconscious. Cool right? But how do we do this? Well, that's exactly what we are going to uncover in the next set of exercises.

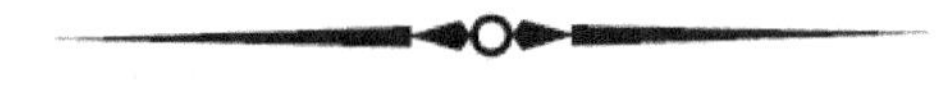

Lucid Dreaming: Exercises for Self-Discovery

Let's now unlock the door to the mysterious world of lucid dreaming, where the boundaries of reality blur, and your subconscious mind takes center stage.

1. Reality Checks: Awake Within the Dream

(ad-hoc)

- Develop a routine of reality checks throughout your day. Engage in mindfulness by questioning your reality, examining details, and performing small tasks like counting fingers. This habit will naturally extend into your dreams, triggering awareness. For example, ask yourself, "Am I dreaming?" and sincerely assess your surroundings.

2. Dream Journals: The Architect's Blueprint

(ad-hoc)

- Always keep a separate dream journal by your bedside within easy reach. As you wake from each dream, capture down on paper all the vivid details – sights, sounds, and emotions. This practice not only enhances your ability to recall dreams but also serves as a map, helping you identify recurring themes related to self-sabotage. Pay attention to the emotions that you feel in your dreams, as they often mirror waking emotions.

3. Set Intentions Before Sleep: Plant the Seeds of Awareness

(2 minutes)

- Before drifting into slumber, set a clear intention to become aware of your dreams. Visualize yourself recognizing the dream state and asserting control. You can do this by repeating to yourself phrases such as "I will be aware that I'm dreaming". This mantra will reinforce your commitment to lucidity, acting as a beacon within your dream world. This pre-sleep ritual will also significantly influence your dream experiences.

4. Visualization: Scripting Your Dream Reality

(2 minutes)

- Engage in visualization exercises before falling asleep. Picture yourself within a dream, confidently facing your self-sabotaging scenarios. Envision moments of resilience and success aligned with your aspirations. This mental rehearsal sets the stage for empowered dreaming. Visualize specific scenarios where you conquer self-sabotage tendencies alongside the specific decision-making need that is foremost in your mind. This will create a dream script, outlining the issue at hand and how you could address various self-sabotage scenarios.

5. Progressive Relaxation: The Gateway to Dream Control

(2 minutes)

- Practice progressive relaxation before bedtime. Systematically tighten and then relax each muscle group, starting from your toes and working your way up to your shoulders and face. Keep on repeating until you begin to feel fully relaxed. This not only induces physical calmness but also prepares your mind for the fluidity of the dream world. Imagine a wave of relaxation sweeping through each part of your body as you repeat the exercise.

6. Explore, Reflect, Empower: The Lucid Dream Walk

(ad-hoc)

- Once within the dream, embrace your role as an active participant in shaping the dream's topic of exploration by referring to your dream script. Confront your fears, practice resilience, and rewrite the narrative of self-sabotage scenarios. Engage with dream characters and dream-created environments consciously rescripting and challenging the situation with various approaches for ever more positive outcomes. Your dreams will become a safe place where you can rehearse approaches and establish favorable outcomes. It will form a canvas for your empowerment.

7. Wake-Back-to-Bed Technique: Navigate the Threshold

(2 minutes)

- Set an alarm to wake you after 4-6 hours of sleep. Upon awakening, engage in a quiet, reflective activity. This brief period of wakefulness disrupts your sleep cycle, making it easier to enter a lucid dream when you return to bed with heightened awareness. Reflect on your dreams during this time, enhancing your connection to your subconscious. Remember to note down any dream experiences that you have had in your dream journal. Include not only what you witnessed, explored, and resolved, but also the feelings that you experienced while doing so.

8. Upon Waking: Record Insights and Patterns

(2 minutes)

- Develop a habit of recording insights immediately upon waking. Note triggers, progress, and recurring patterns related to potential self-sabotage scenarios. This reflective practice transforms your dream experiences into valuable tools for personal growth. Look for connections between dream symbols and real-life situations that trigger your self-sabotage tendencies.

9. Consistency is Key: Cultivate a Lucid Mindset

(Twice per week)

- Lucid dreaming is a hugely valuable skill developed through consistent practice. Try to achieve this state at least twice each week. By implementing these techniques regularly, you will foster a lucid mindset that extends beyond your dreams supporting decision making and action determination in your waking life. Celebrate each step forward on your journey of self-empowerment by noting in your journal which dream-induced decisions have made a positive impact by avoiding self-sabotaging situations.

Navigating your dreamscapes will bring you closer to unveiling the transformative potential that lies within you.

Sweet dreams, fellow traveler.

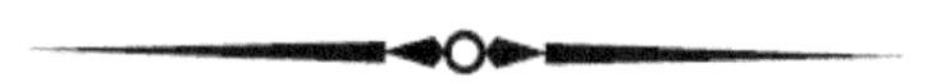

Conclusion: Dreaming as a Catalyst for Transformation

As we conclude this voyage into the dream realm, remember that each night offers you a safe place for self-discovery. Dreams are the whispers of your soul and offer guidance for those on the path to overcoming self-sabotage tendencies. A world that allows you to safely try out new approaches, to discover new, more favorable outcomes empowering your daytime decision-making.

Embrace your nightly dream-shaping, by decoding the symbolism, and letting the landscapes of your dreams become the backdrop for your transformative journey.

In our next leg of the journey, we'll delve into the realm of self-reflection and acceptance, peeling back the layers that cloak our true selves. Until then, may your awareness be your guiding star, illuminating the path to self-discovery.

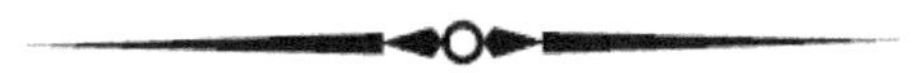

Chapter 3: Embracing Self-Reflection and Acceptance

"No amount of self-improvement can make up for any lack of self-acceptance." [1]

Embrace Knowing Yourself

Welcome, to the truly transformative realm of self-reflection and acceptance, where the power to overcome

---

1. Robert Holden, 2011, "Shift Happens!: How to Live an Inspired Life...Starting Right Now!"

self-sabotage begins with acknowledging without judgment.

Acceptance is a hard thing to conquer but together we will not only learn to gain a far deeper understanding of ourselves but to welcome that knowledge and use it to shape alternative, more positive outcomes. By doing so we will not only cultivate self-compassion but also unravel the intricacies of our vulnerabilities to help avoid self-sabotage situations altogether.

Acceptance through Self-Reflection and Observation

In the following sections, I will first go through the opportunities for self-improvement and then detail the related exercises that can help you bring these into reality

Understanding Self-Sabotage Without Judgment

I am leading in with some nifty painting analogies to bring this topic to life.

Picture this: a canvas painted with the hues of all your experiences, each stroke a reflection of your journey to date. As we dive deep into the world of self-reflection, it's crucial to approach the canvas of self-sabotage without the harsh brush of judgment. Simply acknowledging the patterns, the triggers, and the moments of surrender to self-defeating behaviors will aid you significantly. It's not about blame, it's about creating deep-seated understanding one great brush stroke at a time.

Encouraging Vulnerability Through Self-Reflection

Self-reflection is the mirror that unveils our vulnerabilities, those raw, unfiltered aspects of ourselves that often lie hidden in the shadows where we do our best to avoid them. However here we will actively seek to embrace the understanding of our vulnerabilities as a source of strength, not weakness. By the end of this Chapter, through guided introspection, you will be able to safely explore the roots of your self-sabotage, tracing the threads to their origin without fear or recrimination. It's in these moments of revealed vulnerability that true acceptance begins to take shape and your transformation begins.

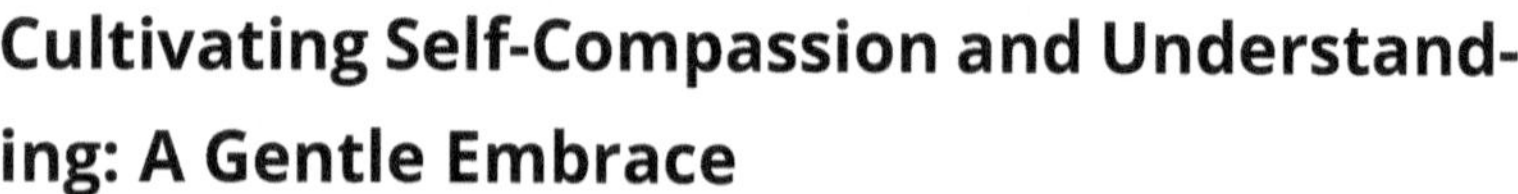

Cultivating Self-Compassion and Understanding: A Gentle Embrace

Techniques for Fostering Self-Compassion

In the tapestry of self-discovery, self-compassion is the golden thread that connects understanding and acceptance. Introduce yourself to the art of self-compassion through mindfulness exercises, affirmations, and self-love practices. Treat yourself with the kindness and understanding you readily offer others and know that you are fully deserving. This is not a journey of perfection but a means of embracing your imperfections like an old friend with open arms.

Addressing Guilt and Shame: The Path to Self-Forgiveness

Guilt and shame often cast long shadows on our path to acceptance. Let's expose them by shining a light into these murky pools of shade enabling us to face them head-on. Acknowledge the heavy weight that they bear upon you, dissecting the layers of self-blame that knit together like a shroud of loathing. Through therapeutic exercises and affirmations, you can release the burdens of guilt and shame that you carry. Self-forgiveness is not a destination but a continuous journey to enable growth and change. Understand that your personal growth will stem from lessons learned, not from the weight of held regret.

Case Studies and Personal Transformations: Stories of Triumph and Renewal

Let's examine real-world narratives of individuals who faced the grip of self-sabotage and emerged victorious. These stories are not just tales but living proof that acceptance is the gateway to transformation. Walk alongside people who navigated their vulnerabilities, embraced self-compassion, and emerged far stronger for it. Their journeys serve as beacons, illuminating the way forward.

Case Study 1: Sara's Turning Point

Sara, a successful marketing manager, found herself trapped in a cycle of perfectionism and constant self-critique. This impacted her levels of acceptance of others whose work would contribute to her own. She was widely known as an exceptionally difficult person to please which impacted her work relationships as a consequence. As her perfectionism grew she began to experience panic attacks and was forever racing against expiring deadlines to submit her work. Through guided self-reflection exercises, she began to acknowledge her deep-rooted fear of failure. Cultivating self-compassion allowed her to face her vulnerabilities without judgment. As she embraced acceptance, Sara discovered a renewed sense of confidence that enabled her to move away from perfectionism and unreachable standards, thereby transforming both her professional and personal life for the better.

Case Study 2: James's Journey to Self-Forgiveness

James, an aspiring artist, struggled with crippling self-doubt and feelings of inadequacy. This led to several bouts of creative block and a severe lack of productivity. The self-reflection exercises led him to safely explore the roots of his negative self-perception. By addressing the guilt and shame associated with his perceived failures, James learned to forgive himself. This act of self-forgiveness became a pivotal moment, unlocking his creative potential that led to a series of successful exhibitions of his work.

Case Study 3: Maria's Resilience Unleashed

Maria faced challenges in her relationships due to her tendency to self-sabotage. Many relationships were short-lived and destined to fall apart based on a lack of trust and moments of extremely controlling behavior. Through the lens of self-reflection, she uncovered the emotional scars from past experiences that affected how she viewed each new relationship. Guided exercises in cultivating self-compassion allowed her to confront and heal those wounds, locking them firmly in the past. Maria's journey became a testament to resilience, illustrating how acceptance can transform pain into strength, ultimately fostering healthier connections and in her case longer, more fulfilling relationships.

Turning Points and Revelations: A Holistic Expedition into Transformation

The narratives shared above from real people illuminate the extraordinary potential of critical turning points in our lives and the need to nurture the circumstances that form them – profound moments driven by a deep understanding of oneself. Now, let's embark on a similar transformative journey by cultivating pathways of self-reflection and compassion that go beneath the surface.

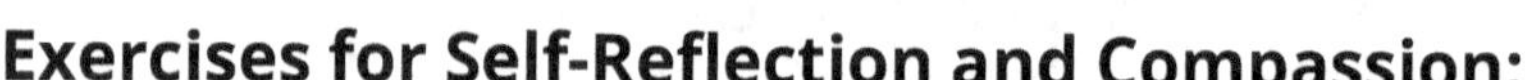

Exercises for Self-Reflection and Compassion:

Below I have listed no fewer than eight exercises designed to support self-reflection and personal compassion. Now I don't expect you to carry out all eight, simply select the ones that work best for you. Remember that their purpose is to develop an actionable framework to help you explore deep inside yourself to unmask the root causes of your self-sabotage. It's important to have an open mind to discover which works best for you as everyone is different and responds to different stimuli to reach the same transformational result.

1. Guided Journaling for Profound Self-Reflection

(20 minutes)

Dive into the depths of your being through the immersive practice of guided journaling. This isn't a casual jotting down of thoughts on the back of a fag packet; it's an intentional exploration of the intricate layers that serve to conceal self-sabotage. Craft questions that are both probing and compassionate, encouraging a dialogue with your inner self. Your journal will transform into a sacred space, a confidant ready to accompany you through the labyrinth of your thoughts and emotions. Embrace any vulnerabilities that you uncover along the way with your internalized questioning as you navigate the "whys" and "hows" of things. Write down your questions and responses and celebrate the complexity of your journey with each pen stroke.

Setting the Scene for Exploration:

1. **Intentional Journaling:** Go beyond casual thoughts; set a clear intention for unraveling self-sabotage complexities.

2. **Crafting Probing Questions:** Formulate compassionate yet probing questions to delve into the "whys" and "hows" of your tendencies.

Journal as a Sacred Space:

1. **JournalTransformation:** Witness your journal becoming a safe repository for your innermost thoughts, a confidant supporting you to gain insights into the twists and turns of your life.

2. **Navigating Vulnerabilities:** Remember to embrace your vulnerabilities without judgment, celebrating their honesty.

Dialogue with Your Inner Self:

1. **Written Conversations:** Engage in written dialogue, exploring hidden layers and gaining insights into self-sabotage patterns.

2. **Celebrating Complexity:** Each question and response celebrates the intricate mosaic of your self-discovery journey as you reveal in ever more detail the reasons behind your self-destructive tendencies.

Conclusion of the Journaling Session:

Ensure that you spend quality time reviewing and reflecting upon the insights gained, as your intentional journaling entries become a set of waypoints, guiding you through self-sabotage with increased self-awareness.

2. Mindfulness Meditation: Cultivating Self-Compassion

(10 minutes)

Immerse yourself in purposeful mindfulness meditations designed to cultivate a rich garden of self-compassion. Find a tranquil space, free from distractions, relax fully, and let the gentle guidance lead you into a state of serene introspection. In these moments, extend genuine kindness to yourself. Recognize that imperfections are not blemishes but integral threads woven into the fabric of the human experience. Everyone has them and you are no different from those around you. Search deep within yourself seeking answers to the feelings that you experience when moments of self-destruction are present. Understand what makes you react in the way you do. As you embrace these imperfections, you are laying the foundation for acceptance and, consequently, the groundwork for transformation.

Guided Meditation for Self-Compassion:

1. **Guided Beginnings:** Start the meditation with this gentle guidance. Focus on your breath, letting each deep inhale and exhale draw you ever deeper into the present moment. As you center yourself, let your thoughts guide you toward self-compassion. Examine past situations where self-sabotage occurred and the circumstances around them in a passive non-confrontational manner.

2. **Extending Genuine Kindness:** In these moments of mindful introspection, extend genuine kindness to yourself. Recognize that imperfections are not flaws but integral aspects of the shared human experience. Understand that, just like those around you, you carry the tapestry of imperfections that make you beautifully unique.

Deep Dive into Self-Reflection:

1. **Seeking Answers Within:** During this meditation, enter the depths of your being. Explore the feelings that surface when moments of self-sabotage cast their shadows from your memory. Uncover the triggers and reactions, understanding the intricacies of your emotional landscape.

2. **Understanding Reactions:** As you navigate this in-

ternal terrain, seek understanding. What lies beneath the surface of your reactions? What past experiences or beliefs influence the way you respond to such challenges? This introspective journey is a pivotal step toward unraveling the roots of your self-sabotage.

Conclusion of the Meditation:

As you conclude this mindfulness meditation, linger in the serene afterglow. Let the echoes of self-compassion reverberate through your being. This practice serves to cultivate self-understanding and acceptance. The seeds of transformative growth have been planted, and with each meditative journey, you nurture the flourishing landscape of self-compassion.

3. Letter to Your Past Self: Crafting Compassion

(30 minutes)

In this deeply introspective exercise, you are invited to pick up pen and paper and write a letter to the version of yourself that once danced to the rhythm of questionable fashion and cringy music. Yes, your younger self. This exercise isn't just about acknowledging moments tainted by self-sabotage; it's an act of self-understanding and compassion. This exercise is best approached with an open heart, free from judgment, seeking to learn from the truth that led to the circumstances of your past life. Offer words of comfort, understanding, and encouragement. This letter will serve as a symbolic bridge, connecting the chapters of your past to the narrative of your present. It's an intimate act of self-forgiveness and acceptance.

The Art of Compassionate Reflection:

1. **Setting the Scene:** Find a tranquil space where you can immerse yourself in this introspective journey. Light a candle, play soft music, or surround yourself with comforting scents, whichever works for you in creating an environment conducive to self-reflection.

2. **Open-Hearted Beginnings:** As you start the letter, approach it with genuine kindness, free from the constraints of judgment. Visualize your past self with a caring, compassionate gaze, recognizing the circumstances, challenges, and triumphs that shaped that unique chapter of your life.

3. **Acknowledging Imperfections:** Reflect on those moments of your life that you wish to comment on. The decisions made and later regretted, those sacrificed ideals that never got picked back up. Embrace the imperfections of your past self with considered tenderness. Understand that each choice, even those tainted by self-sabotage, was a part of your evolution to the present day.

4. **Words of Comfort and Understanding:** Offer sincere words of comfort, understanding, and encour-

agement to your past self. Speak to them as you would a dear friend who experienced the same trials. Share insights gained through present-day wisdom, extending a hand of reassurance.

Conclusion of the Exercise:

As you conclude your soul-stirring letter, bask in the resonance of self-understanding and compassion. This exercise serves to connect the dots between your past and present self. It supports realization and change, nurturing the seeds of self-forgiveness and acceptance. In crafting this intimate letter, you honor the journey that shaped you, integrating the past into the evolving narrative of your present.

4. Reflective Dialogue with Inner Archetypes: Unmasking the Voices Within

(10 minutes)

Engage in a reflective dialogue with your inner archetypes – those subconscious facets that influence your thoughts and behaviors. Personify them, assigning each archetype a distinct identity. Initiate a conversation, allowing them to express themselves. This exercise unveils the dynamics playing out within your psyche, shedding light on the origins of your self-sabotage. As you unravel these intricate layers, you empower yourself to navigate challenges with newfound wisdom and self-awareness.

Examples of Inner Archetypes:

1. **The Protector:** This archetype may manifest as a stern, vigilant guardian within you. It often surfaces in moments of perceived threat or vulnerability, acting as a shield against potential harm. Engaging in a dialogue with your Protector may reveal insights into the origins of self-sabotage, unveiling patterns established as defense mechanisms.

2. **The Critic:** This internal voice tends to be hypercritical, setting unrealistically high standards and fostering self-doubt that you will never achieve them. Personifying the Critic allows you to understand its motivations and origins. Through conversation, you may uncover the roots of ingrained beliefs contributing to self-sabotage, offering an opportunity for compassionate resolution.

3. **The Nurturer:** This archetype embodies compassion and care, and is often overshadowed by louder, more critical voices. By personifying the Nurturer, you can explore how this aspect of yourself responds to moments of self-sabotage. Understanding its presence allows you to cultivate self-compassion, creating a harmonious balance within.

4. **The Rebel:** Sometimes, an inner Rebel emerges, challenging established norms and seeking autonomy through extreme and daring actions. Through dialogue, you may uncover the Rebel's motivations,

exploring whether self-sabotage is a form of subconscious resistance. This awareness opens avenues for constructive alignment of your desires and actions.

Here's how to Engage in Reflective Dialogue:

1. **Identification:** Begin by identifying the dominant archetypes within you. Reflect on moments when certain patterns, thoughts, or emotions emerge consistently. Do you listen more to the snide remarks of the Critic or follow the extreme advice of the Rebel inside?

2. **Visualization:** Create mental images that represent each archetype. Picture their appearance, demeanor, and unique characteristics. Visualizing them in this manner aids in making your dialogue with them more vivid and real.

3. **Initiate Conversation:** Choose a quiet, contemplative space where you will not be disturbed. Mentally address each archetype, inviting them to share their perspectives. You might say, "Protector, I acknowledge your presence. What are your concerns?" Allow each archetype to respond.

4. **Active Listening:** Practice active listening within your mind. Pay attention to the nuances of each archetype's responses. Note any emotions, memories, or insights that surface during your dialogue.

5. **Record Insights:** Use your journal to capture the insights gained during the conversation. Note the origins of specific archetypes, their roles in your life, and how they have contributed to or hindered your actions of the past and present.

Conclusion of the Dialogue:

As you engage in this reflective dialogue, you are effectively peeling back the layers of your psyche, revealing the intricate interconnection of your inner archetypes and your motivations and resultant behaviors. By understanding their distinct motivations, you gain insight into the origins of your self-sabotage. This exercise empowers you to navigate life's challenges with newfound self-awareness and wisdom, fostering a harmonious and balanced integration of these subconscious facets on your driving forces and decision-making rationale.

5. Vision Board Creation for Future Alignment

(30 -60 minutes)

Oh Yes, we had to get to your creative self. For this exercise, I want you to unleash your inner artist as you embark on a creative journey to shape your destiny through the practice of crafting a vision board. This isn't merely about your aspirations but a focused alignment with your authentic self, bringing your future self into focus. Here's how to make your vision board a dynamic and evolving guide on your path of transformation.

Collective Ingredients for Alignment:

1. **Selecting Evocative Imagery:** Choose images that deeply resonate with your personal goals, values, and authentic self. These can take the form of photos' magazine cuttings or digital elements if you wish to use a digital canvas for your endeavors.

2. **Words as Anchors:** Incorporate powerful words, quotes, and phrases that anchor your vision, reinforcing your path of self-acceptance.

3. **Symbols of Significance:** Integrate symbols representing pivotal aspects of your journey toward self-acceptance and transformation. These could be drawn or photographed or even stuck on if you are a creative type.

Creation Process and Unveiling Potential:

1. **Crafting the Visual Collage:** Organize your chosen elements into a visually compelling collage, creating a story of your envisioned future. This should reflect your desired state after overcoming your self-sabotaging tendencies. It should also show how you understand your past emotional and physical drivers and how you will overcome them to form new more positive outcomes. This is in effect determining the vision you have of the person you want to be. Your future self with all the attributes that you hold dear and none of the ones you see as negative

or inhibiting.

2. **Daily Reminder Effect:** Position your vision board in a prominent place for daily viewing, allowing it to serve as a potent reminder of your transformative journey ahead.

3. **Regular Revisiting and Rejuvenation:** Periodically (possibly monthly) revisit and update your vision board to reflect the evolving chapters of your self-acceptance and transformation. Feel the emotional resonance as you connect with the vivid representations of your journey, reinforcing your commitment to change to become the person that you wish to be.

Conclusion of the Vision Board Journey:

Regularly immerse yourself in the living visual narrative of your vision board, letting it guide your steps toward alignment with your authentic self. Celebrate each update as a testament to your evolving self-acceptance and the transformative path that you are on.

6. Gratitude Journaling for Positive Reinforcement

(10 minutes)

Elevate your daily routine with the transformative power of gratitude journaling, a practice that goes beyond mere acknowledgment to become a profound source of positive reinforcement. Here's how to infuse your life with gratitude, gradually diminishing the shadows of self-sabotage and nurturing inner strength and resilience.

Initiating the Gratitude Ritual:

1. **Daily Moments of Appreciation:** Cultivate the habit of identifying and recording moments of joy, accomplishment, and personal growth daily. This can be through setting aside a specific time to capture your thoughts or by capturing them on the fly as they happen. Use whichever method works for you.

2. **Reflective Acknowledgment:** Delve into the depth of your experiences, acknowledging not just the obvious triumphs but the subtle victories that often escape notice. Several minor events can make for a big win.

Shifting Perspectives and Diminishing Shadows:

1. **Focus on the Positive:** Weave a tapestry of positivity by directing your focus towards the bright threads of gratitude which will serve over time to alter your perspective on life.

2. **Gradual Erosion of Self-Sabotage:** As gratitude becomes a consistent repeatable theme, you'll witness the gradual erosion of the power self-sabotage has over your mindset. Finding and celebrating be-

comes a habit-forming practice for all those neurons floating about in your brain-shaped computer. The more that those little fella's recognize the importance of positive events and decision-making the more they will encourage it. A virtual circle of positivity all in a head-shaped space.

Cultivating a Positive Mindset:

1. **Mindful Reflection:** Engage in mindful reflection as you write down your positive gratitude statements, savoring each moment and allowing that gratitude to permeate your consciousness.

2. **Resilience Building:** Transform your mindset by actively acknowledging these positives, fostering resilience in the face of future challenges.

Empowerment Through Gratitude:

1. **Positive Affirmations:** Transform your journal into a repository of positive affirmations, reinforcing your self-empowerment journey.

2. **Periodic Review and Celebration:** Periodically review your gratitude journal, celebrating the evolving chapters of your positivity and personal growth. By reassessing what you have written and experiencing those positive feelings anew you are strengthening the habit-forming bond of positive recognition, training those super-happy neurons to look for ever more positive outcomes for your fu-

ture interactions. Exciting stuff!

Conclusion of Gratitude Journaling Journey:

By making gratitude gathering a daily ritual, you're not just documenting moments; you're crafting a narrative of positivity and self-empowerment. Watch as your gratitude journal becomes a testament to your resilience, diminishing the influence of self-sabotage, and paving the way for habit-forming growth.

7. Inner Child Visualization: Nurturing Healing

(10 minutes)

Embark on a profound inner child visualization journey, delving into the depths of your psyche to connect with and nurture your far younger self. This transformative exercise is designed to provide a compassionate space for healing, addressing unmet needs from the past and unveiling hidden drivers of self-sabotage tendencies.

Initiating the Inner Child Journey:

1. **Create a Tranquil Space:** Set the stage for your visualization in a calm and serene environment, free from distractions and interruptions.

2. **Relaxation Techniques:** Engage in relaxation techniques, such as deep breathing or progressive muscle relaxation, to ease into a state conducive to visualization.

Encountering Your Inner Child:

1. **Visualize Your Younger Self:** In this relaxed state, visualize encountering your inner child. Picture the younger version of yourself, perhaps at a pivotal age where certain experiences left a lasting impact.

2. **Create a Safe Space:** Envision a safe and nurturing space where you can interact with your inner child without judgment or inhibition.

Offering Comfort and Reassurance:

1. **Comforting Dialogue:** Engage in a comforting dialogue with your inner child, offering reassurance, love, and understanding. Address any specific memories or emotions that surface.

2. **Identifying Unmet Needs:** Explore any unmet needs from your past that may be contributing to your self-sabotaging tendencies of today. This is a crucial step in unearthing the root causes of your behavioral patterns. Were there specific situations that shaped certain behaviors such as self-protection or aggression? Have these occurrences transformed into inner voices or archetypes that shape your responses to certain situations today? Explore these with sensitivity and remember to capture them down for later reflection.

Fostering Healing and Compassion:

1. **Symbolic Gestures:** Use symbolic gestures, such as embracing or comforting your inner child, to symbolize your commitment to healing and self-acceptance.

2. **Nurturing Relationships:** Visualize building a nurturing relationship with your inner child, fostering a sense of safety and trust within yourself.

Contributing to Self-Acceptance:

1. **Reflective Journaling:** After the visualization, engage in reflective journaling to capture insights, emotions, and any newfound self-awareness. Consider how the encounter with your inner child influences your perception of self-sabotage events both past and current.

2. **Integrate Learnings:** Integrate the learnings from this visualization into your daily life, recognizing and addressing patterns that may be rooted in unmet childhood needs. Embrace the ongoing process of self-acceptance and transformation as you continue to nurture and support your relationship with your inner child.

8. Personal Mantra Development for Empowerment

(10 minutes)

Develop a personal mantra that encapsulates strength, resilience, and self-empowerment based on your uncovered learnings. Craft a phrase or affirmation that strongly resonates with your journey toward overcoming self-sabotage. Repeat this mantra regularly, especially during more challenging moments. The mantra serves as a powerful tool to rewire your thought patterns and reinforce a positive mindset, becoming an anchor in your pursuit of transformation and changed outcomes.

Embark on Your Persoformation

These exercises serve not merely as tasks to complete but gateways to self-revelation, each offering a unique perspective into the intricate landscape of your psyche. With warm encouragement, begin your transformation by engaging with the exercises that work for you consistently, allowing them to serve as companions on your journey toward self-discovery, acceptance, and renewal.

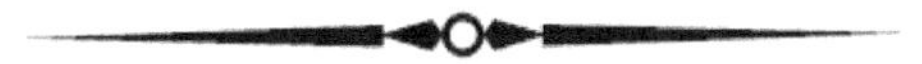

Chapter 4: Understanding Emotional Wounds

"Healing may not be so much about getting better, as about letting go of everything that isn't you – all of the expectations, all of the beliefs – and becoming who you are." [1]

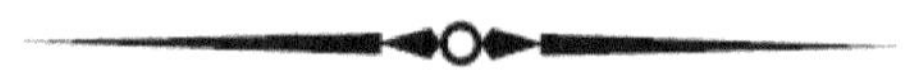

Dear Readers,

As we navigate the intricate inner expedition of self-discovery, our compass unfailingly directs us toward the realm of emotional wounds – those concealed scars of the past that linger well into our present, steering us toward self-sabo-

---

1.

taging behavior. These are the wounds that cut deep, causing anguish at the time and, for some inexplicable reason, endure taunting us from beneath our skin. That painful breakup, those schoolyard beatings, the parental abuse – these experiences can remain with you, casting a lingering shadow over your behaviors. Each scar infects us at certain moments in our lives with negative intent that harms our potential. To forge a path toward transformation, we must delve deep within ourselves, unraveling the threads that tie our past wounds to our present behaviors and learn how to heal the emotional scars that fuel our self-destructive tendencies.

Exploring Emotional Triggers and Past Wounds:

Our journey commences with a tender exploration of the emotional triggers entwined with our self-sabotage tendencies. These triggers often have roots in our past, wounds that may have been overlooked but continue to influence our present-day choices. Let us look into the significance of these triggers, and understand how they perpetuate patterns of self-destructive behaviors that negatively impact our lives.

Allow me to share a personal anecdote to illuminate these concepts. Despite external success, I never felt truly worthy. This broad yet profound sentiment, rooted in years of being put down and made to feel like a failure, impacted my emotional state and my personal and business relationships. Recognizing these emotional triggers and understanding their origins allowed me to navigate the path of healing. By acknowledging past wounds, and their power over us we empower ourselves to break free from their shackles.

Addressing Past Wounds:

Our personal histories are intricate stories, each page narrating a tale of triumphs and tribulations. To comprehend the connection between past wounds and self-sabotage, approach these memories with gentle curiosity. Allow the narrative of your life to unfold, exposing moments of vulnerability, hurt, and resilience. Traverse the landscapes of your past, paying particular attention to pivotal events that may have etched deep imprints into your beliefs.

Simultaneously, turn your gaze toward emotional triggers that act as silent orchestrators of self-sabotage. Immerse yourself in your emotional backstory, exploring the minutiae of situations, interactions, or feelings that are still evoking intense responses. Is it the echoes of criticism, the lingering taste of rejection, or the looming specter of failure that is triggering your self-destructive tendencies?

Identifying these triggers is the first and most important empowering step toward conscious navigation.

Exercise: Guided Journaling for Profound Exploration

To embark on this exercise, create a dedicated section in your journal. This is a sacred space where with each stroke of the pen you explore deeper into the recesses of your past. As you seek out these past life moments you will unearth memories, emotions, and patterns of behavior that have traveled with you throughout your personal history.

Consider the real impact of significant life events – both joyous and challenging – on your self-perception. Invite introspection into how these events might have left imprints on your beliefs, influencing the choices that you make and the way you view the world. This journal is not merely a collection of words but a living archive, a potent tool for unraveling the threads that bind past wounds to present behaviors.

As you undertake this journaling expedition, remember that your story is a personal history ingrained with resilience, vulnerability, and growth.

Healing Inner Emotional Scars and Trauma

Embarking on the journey of healing our inner emotional scars and traumas requires a nuanced understanding and deliberate, compassionate practices. Let's explore strategies for emotional healing with a depth that transcends surface feelings, recognizing that each emotional scar is a chapter in our personal epic novel.

Strategies for Emotional Healing:

Imagine that your emotional scars are a testament to your resilience and fortitude over all the years of your life. These scars are not blemishes but entries etched deep into your being. To foster emotional healing, we must embark on a journey of self-compassion. This involves embracing mindfulness as a guiding philosophy, weaving self-care rituals into your daily routine, and forging connections with trusted individuals who can provide you with unwavering support.

Acknowledge that healing is not a hurried activity but an organic process that may take time to complete. This time will be time well spent. It also requires patience, gentleness, and a commitment to honoring the emotions that arise along the way. Simply burying unwelcome past situations and their impact on your emotional being is no good. It's like burying treasure, someone will come along and dig it up again. As you take this journey, consider seeking professional guidance if needed, recognizing that external support can be a valuable signpost on the path to healing.

Resilience-Building:

Resilience is the bullet-proof vest that shields us from life's gunshot wounds, and intentionally building this armor is paramount, especially if you happen to live in a rough neighborhood. Strengthen the core of your being through deliberate practices that go beyond the conventional boundaries of physical well-being and explore emotional health and resilience. Engage also in regular physical exercise, not just as a routine but as a conscious act of fortifying your body as well as your mind. You want to be fit on the outside as well as on the inside.

Fortifying the Core: A Holistic Approach

Physical and mental well-being is the foundation upon which your resilience will be built. Let's now explore some of the practices that you can undertake to fortify your core.

Exercise 1: Physical Empowerment Routine

(30 minutes)

Design a personalized exercise routine that blends cardiovascular activities, strength training, and flexibility exercises. Tailor it to your preferences, ensuring it serves as a holistic approach to your physical well-being. If you are not confident in designing this process then seek the help of a dedicated physical trainer. These guys and girls can build out a bespoke routine that meets your individual needs. Ensure that you follow through by exercising if not daily then every second day. Your confidence will grow as you see physical progress being made.

Immersing in the Present: Mindfulness Exploration

Mindfulness practices serve as the anchor, grounding us in the present moment amidst life's headwinds. It's not just a passing trend; it's a profound practice enabling the cultivation of resilience by navigating challenges with both clarity and poise.

Exercise 2: Crafting Your Mindful Exercise - A Comprehensive Mindful Moments Journal

(30 minutes)

In this journey of mindfulness, creating a "Mindful Moments" journal section transcends mere documentation; it becomes a sacred chronicle of your evolving relationship with the present.

1. **Setting the Scene: A Mindful Journal Sanctuary**
   Begin by dedicating a special journal or a digital space exclusively for your mindful moments. This act is symbolic, signifying the sacredness of your mindfulness exploration.

2. **Embark on Daily Mindful Quests**
   Each day, embark on intentional quests to notice and acknowledge moments of mindfulness. These can range from the simple act of savoring your

morning coffee to the complex yet beautiful interplay of nature during an evening walk.

3. **Chronicle Multifaceted Moments**

Document your experiences with a poetic touch. Describe not only the external circumstances but delve into the internal landscape – the sensations, emotions, and thoughts that accompany each mindful moment.

4. **Reflections on Resilience**

After recording your mindful moments, engage in reflective sessions. Consider how each instance contributes to your mental resilience. Explore the subtle shifts in your perception, emotional regulation, and overall well-being.

5. **Building Themes and Patterns**

Over time, notice emerging themes and patterns in your mindful moments. Are there specific activities, environments, or people that consistently anchor you in the present? Understanding these patterns adds depth to your mindfulness practice.

6. **Interactive Mindfulness Mapping**

Create visual representations or mind maps that showcase the interconnected web of your mindful moments. This visual exploration enhances your understanding of the intricate relationship between mindfulness and your resilience.

Mindful journaling becomes a comforting companion, capturing the essence of your evolving relationship with the present, fostering resilience, and contributing to your transformative journey.

Valued Human Connections

Human connections are the bedrock of who we are and who we try to be. They act as trusted supportive comrades when chosen well. Actively seek out a supportive community that aligns with your values and aspirations. These connections become the reinforcement that strengthens your resilience.

Exercise 3: Building a Resilience Network

(Variable)

Identify individuals in your life who contribute positively to your well-being. Foster deeper connections with them, whether through regular conversations, shared activities, or mutual support. Build out a network that serves as a resilient foundation in your times of need. Think of the AA support network as a prime example. Each person looks after the other in some way either by communicating their back story, confiding in their needs, celebrating triumphs, or directly acting as a mentor and support to others when times are tough.

Remember, resilience is not just about enduring; it's about thriving in the face of challenges. With a fortified core, anchored presence, and supportive connections, you are cultivating a robust resilience that will empower you to face life's uncertainties with renewed strength.

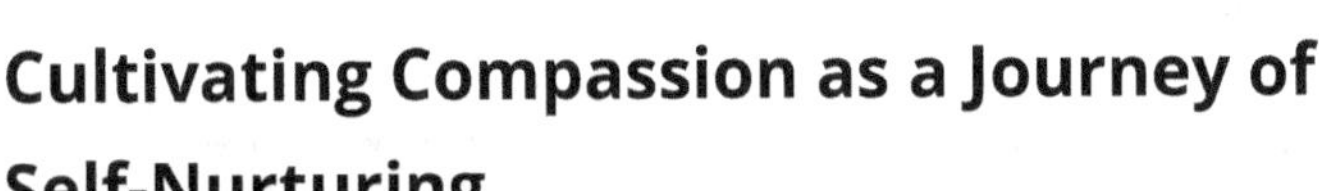

Cultivating Compassion as a Journey of Self-Nurturing

Self-compassion is akin to a gentle summer breeze. It is the balm that hastens the healing process, tenderly anointing emotional wounds. It's an internal dialogue bathed in kindness, a recognition that imperfections are not flaws but unique facets of your humanity. To foster this self-nurturing discourse, we need to enter the depths of compassionate self-talk that effortlessly counters the bellowing shouts of self-criticism with waves of gentle encouragement.

Exercise: Affirmations as a Self-Compassion Daily Ritual

(10 minutes)

Affirmation Elixir

Begin this exercise by crafting affirmations that resonate with the very essence of your healing journey. These will not be merely words but powerful personal indictments of compassion. They are the potent elixirs of positivity and resilience, each phrase carefully chosen to resonate with your soul. Swallow this medicine at least twice a day, ideally with a good meal. Remember that crafting affirmations is a deeply personal process, and the examples provided below are only meant to inspire and guide you in creating affirmations that resonate with your unique journey of healing and self-compassion:

I am deserving of love, kindness, and understanding.

My past does not define me; I am creating a future full of strength and resilience.

Each step forward is a victory, a testament to my courage and tenacity.

I forgive myself for past mistakes and welcome the wisdom they've bestowed.

Every breath I take, every move forward I make, fills me with renewed energy and positivity.

Whatever form your affirmations take be sure to make them uniquely personal and powerful for you. Use your self-awareness and insight so far gained to make them drivers for a change in mindset.

A Daily Ritual, Not a Routine

Immerse yourself in the affirmations daily, but with inten-tionality. This isn't a mechanical routine like flossing but a sacred ritual, a moment carved out for the communion of your inner self. Engage in this ritual with mindfulness, allowing each affirmation to permeate your consciousness.

1. **The Power of Repetition**

   Repetition is the key to embedding these affirmations into the fabric of your thoughts. Repeat them with conviction, not as a monotonous chant, but as a symphony, each repetition building upon the last forming a crescendo of self-compassion within.

2. **Visual Reinforcement**

   Enhance the impact by complementing verbal recitation with visual reinforcement. Create visual displays of your affirmations – perhaps a vision board or strategically placed notes or items of emotional value. Visual cues serve to reinforce the positive narrative, acting as constant reminders of your ultimate strength and worthiness.

3. **Affirmation Journaling**

   Maintain an affirmation section in your journal to capture the evolving dynamics of your self-talk. Document how these affirmations influence your emotions, reactions, and overall well-being. Reflect on the subtle shifts and celebrate new milestones.

Introduction to Therapeutic Practices and Self-Healing Techniques

In the realm of emotional exploration, professional counseling often offers valuable guidance. A therapist provides a safe space, tools, insights, and an empathetic presence. Incorporating therapeutic techniques into your self-healing journeys, such as guided imagery, expressive arts, and cognitive-behavioral exercises can aid the process. Embrace these practices as channels for creative exploration and self-discovery.

In concluding this chapter, let your journey of understanding emotional wounds guide you toward self-discovery and healing. Use the insights gained and the practices embraced here to lead you to a future imbued with resilience, self-compassion, and positive transformation.

Chapter 5: Shifting Limiting Beliefs

"Whether you think you can, or you think you can't—you're right." [1]

As we continue our journey of self-discovery, we now set our sights on the formidable land of limiting beliefs. These are the invisible chains that contain and control our potential, the whispered doubts that echo in the deep recesses of our minds. In this chapter, we embark on exploring and challenging these negative beliefs, initiating a profound mindset shift. Together, we will traverse the techniques to conquer self-doubt, reframe limiting beliefs, and cultivate a positive mindset that propels us toward growth and affirmation.

1.

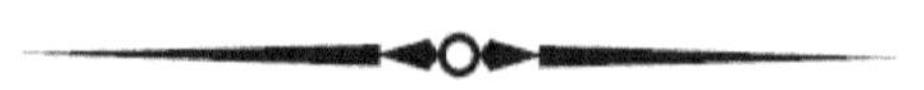

Challenging Negative Beliefs

Our inner dialogue, that constant chatter within our minds, can either be a supportive ally or a relentless adversary. You know the discussions that I am referring to. The ones that can encourage us in every endeavor or sow doubt and fear stopping us in our tracks. This is the double-sided blade of positive and negative self-talk. Unfortunately for many of us, negative self-talk has a far louder voice. "Hey Don't do that, you will fail!", "They all hate what you do, you suck at this job!", or perhaps "They don't love you anymore"; these bear all the attributes of negative self-talk, and let me tell you, all those attributes are bad ones. This insidious creature often inflicts itself upon us at our most anxious moments, making every situation worse and increasing the potential for self-destructive behavior to take place. Negative self-talk is often rooted in what we describe as limiting beliefs and is often a formidable obstacle on the path to personal growth. Let's now take a look at some techniques to challenge this negativity and embark on a journey of mindset transformation.

Techniques to Challenge Negative Self-Talk:

Negative self-talk is like a persistent rain cloud overshadowing our potential. We can be happily walking along and then all of a sudden the sky grows dark and it buckets down before we get the chance to run for cover. I'm English so I always carry an umbrella even on the sunniest of days. So I am in the right place to help you challenge this situation. I'm also quite dry.

To tackle negative self-talk, we must first become aware of its presence. Imagine your mind as a beautiful garden, and your negative thoughts as the pervasive weeds threatening to stifle the life of your vibrant blooms. By acknowledging these weeds, identifying their patterns, and actively challenging their validity you can significantly shift your mindset back to happy, sunny, and flourishing. Let's start with a support mechanism that you may now recognize:

Exercise 1: Thought Recognition Journal

(20 minutes)

Create a "Thought Recognition Journal" to track negative self-talk. Yes, I know that your journal is already looking pretty full by now but hey, buy a bigger one. Whenever a negative thought arises, make sure to jot it down. Note the circumstances, the emotions it creates, and importantly the triggers surrounding it. This journal will become a valuable tool for identifying recurring patterns and for understanding the context in which negative beliefs thrive. No one likes weeks invading their lawn but we need to catch them early to ensure that we are best placed to eradicate them.

OK enough with the garden analogies.

Once you have identified, these negative feelings challenge them with logical counterarguments. For example, if that inner voice whispers, "I am not capable of that," counter it with evidence of your past achievements and capabilities. Perhaps its words tell you that "It's all over in this relationship, you should cut and run". Counter by reflecting on the good times and signs that the relationship is very much alive and well. It's not always as dark and gloomy as negative self-talk would have you believe. Keep on nurturing your more positive inner voices and over time, this practice will weaken the grip that negative beliefs have over you. We are often our own worst enemy, so tell yourself to be kind to you.

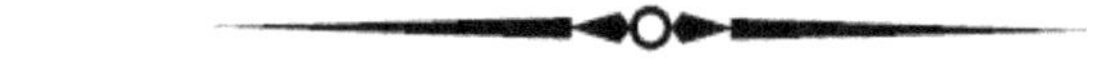

Reframing Limiting Beliefs:

Limiting beliefs are like giant invisible fences, confining us to ever smaller versions of ourselves. The key to dismantling these fences lies in the reframing of our hindering beliefs. Let's now turn our attention to cognitive-behavioral exercises that will facilitate this transformative process.

Introduction to Cognitive-Behavioral Exercises:

Cognitive-behavioral exercises sound pretty psychologically driven, don't they? But at the same time, they are immensely powerful tools for challenging and reshaping our negative thought patterns. The exercises below are designed to explore the intricate connection between our thoughts, our emotions, and our resulting behaviors, offering us a roadmap for a positive shift in mindset.

Exercise 2: The ABC Model - Unraveling Negative Beliefs

(30 minutes)

Welcome to a tried and tested exercise designed to unravel negative beliefs paving the way for a mindset transformation. Let's break it down with simplicity and clarity using the ABC Model. Think of it as your trusty toolkit for cultivating a more positive and balanced you.

A - Activating Event:

The journey begins with identifying the Activating Event, the trigger that sets everything in motion. It could be anything from receiving critical feedback to facing a challenging situation with loved ones. Pinpointing exactly what initiates the chain of negative thoughts and emotions is critical.

B - Belief about the Event:

Next up is "B" for Belief. This represents the actual thoughts and beliefs that automatically surface in response to the Activating Event. Imagine it as the narrative your mind weaves around the situation. Let's say the activating event is receiving critical feedback from your boss, and the belief that follows is *"I am such a failure."*

C - Consequence or Emotional Response:

Now, "C" stands for Consequence, referring to the emotional responses triggered by the belief. In our example, the belief *"I am such a failure"* might lead to feelings of despair and inadequacy. Equally, it could evoke anger or stubbornness in your responses to the feedback. Remember the flight or fight response, well that is all happening in your brain as it figures out how to respond to events and beliefs.

Challenge and Transform:

So now that you have captured the moment or situation and the belief that it triggers as well as your response to that belief, it's time to challenge the outcome. We do that by challenging the irrational beliefs (B). Start this by questioning them. Are they based on facts or merely irrational assumptions? Could there be alternative and more likely and favorable perspectives? For our example, consider acknowledging areas of improvement rather than sticking to the belief of being an overall failure.

Replace with Rational Alternatives:

Now, replace those irrational circumstantial beliefs with more balanced and rational alternatives. If *"I am such a failure"* is the initial belief, transform it into *"I am continuously learning and growing, and there are areas where I can improve."* This shift sets the stage for a more positive and constructive mindset and a better overall response.

Let's examine the example in a bit more detail. You have just run through a presentation with your boss and she has responded quite critically. She dislikes its conclusions and how you have presented the data and wants you to change it. Your initial belief response actively supported by those negative inner voices is that you are a failure. "*You never get the hang of presenting facts and conclusions. Maybe you should look to do something else instead*". Your response would normally be to become angry with yourself and stubborn to any thoughts of a rewrite. However, before you head down that oft-traveled route to antagonizing your boss you instead spend a moment considering some alternatives. Perhaps your boss isn't being mean at all but is actively trying to improve your knowledge and understanding. You start remembering instances where such feedback has enabled you to create better and more accurate presentations which the audience has found really interesting. By accepting this new belief you can receive the feedback more openly and be actively involved in adapting the presentation deck which ultimately improves it. This approach encourages your boss to share further advice and together you create an outstanding piece of work without any antagonization involved.

Remember, these exercises are a dynamic process. It's not about denying your emotions but reshaping the beliefs that drive them. By challenging and transforming negative beliefs, you're taking a proactive step towards fostering a mindset that aligns with your growth and well-being. Go ahead, give it a try, and witness the transformative power of the ABC Model in action.

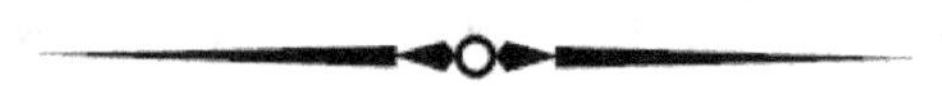

Tools for Positive Growth:

Having confronted your negative beliefs, we now transition to tools that foster a more positive mindset and affirmations for growth. These tools are the seeds we plant in our minds that require nurturing to later blossom into a more resilient and optimistic outlook. OK, that was a string of garden metaphors.. but you get my point. Basically, reap what you sow...

Practical Methods for Fostering a Positive Mindset:

Cultivating a positive mindset requires intentional and consistent effort. If you have been used to limiting yourself by promoting these negative thoughts then it will take some time to junk this bad habit. You have in effect preprogrammed your brain to think that way through long-term acceptance and like any habit it will take patience and determination to overcome it. Just know, that now you are aware of it you can fight it and succeed. And to help you I have included another exercise.

Exercise 3: Gratitude Practice

(30 minutes)

Initiate a daily gratitude practice. Regularly reflect on and list down all the things that you are grateful for that day. It could be the love of your family, a healthy workout, the support of a colleague, or your friends that you meet. This practice redirects focus from what's lacking to what's abundant in your life and abundance is good. It serves as a powerful antidote to negative thinking and fosters a more positive perspective. To do this you should engage regularly in reflective exercises, identifying moments, experiences, or individuals for which you feel genuine gratitude. This daily act of acknowledging and appreciating positive aspects of your life will gradually help to reshape your mindset from negative to positive.

Use this as a daily ritual of acknowledging the richness that life unfolds before us. Here are more details on how to do it.

Initiate Your Gratitude Journey:
Start your day with a moment of reflection. Pause and appreciate the gift of a new day, the warmth of sunlight streaming through your window, or the soothing sounds of nature. This initiation sets the tone for a day infused with gratitude and recognition.

Reflect and List:
Now, let's head into the heart of the exercise with your

trusty journal in hand. Regularly reflect and list all of the things that spark gratitude in your heart. It could be the supportive friends who stood by you, the simple pleasures of a good glass of wine, or the lessons learned from challenges met. The key is to embrace the diversity of gratitude, acknowledging both the grand and the seemingly ordinary.

Beyond the Obvious:

Challenge yourself to move beyond the obvious sources of gratitude. Dig deep into the intricacies of your day. Perhaps it's the unexpected kindness of a stranger or the resilience you displayed during a tough moment. Uncover the layers of gratitude that often go unnoticed when life is a whirlwind of actions and decision-making. Make sure that you note them all down so that you can reflect on them later.

Gratitude Meditation for Mind-Heart Harmony:

Combine gratitude with meditation for a potent fusion of mind-heart harmony. In a quiet space, reflect on the moments of gratitude that you have experienced. Review your journal and relive those diligently captured moments and the emotions that they inspired. Allow these sensations to resonate within you. As you breathe deeply and relax your body let the waves of gratitude permeate every part of your being. This meditation exercise will deepen your connection with positive emotions, paving the way for a shift in your general mindset.

These exercises enable you to undertake practices of gratitude and mindfulness which will guide you toward a mindset infused with positivity, abundance, and an unwavering appreciation for the life you leed.

You may have selected this book because you realized that your life was not going in the direction you wanted. That your self-sabotaging tendencies were taking you to places you didn't want to visit like a lost Uber Driver, however, by undertaking these exercises you may start to realize that not everything is as bad as you think. There is always something good and positive to take away from how your life is progressing, and calling them out is a good way of negating the effects of negative self-talk and limiting belief forming. Know that each moment of gratitude is a step closer to forming a flourishing mindset.

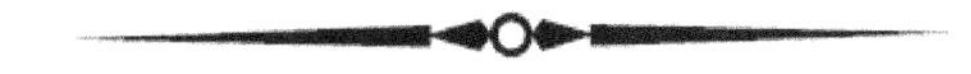

Visualization for Growth

Until now we have spent a lot of time focusing on the past and present so it feels timely to consider the future you instead. Visualization is a technique that involves mentally rehearsing positive outcomes. It's a bit like resealing the envelope around your end-of-year tax demand. It acts as your bridge between the current state and your envisioned future state, facilitating mindset shifts toward growth and affirmation.

Exercise 4: Future Self Visualization

(10 minutes)

Here's an exercise: Close your eyes and visualize your ideal future self. Envision achieving your goals, overcoming challenges, and embodying all of the qualities that you aspire to possess. When attempting to visualize this future self engage your senses – see, hear, and feel the success and growth you desire. If it helps write this down or if you are a creative soul try drawing what represents success for you.

Regularly revisit this mental image, allowing it to shape your beliefs and actions as you intentionally work toward your vision. Visualization enhances motivation, confidence, and resilience, paving the way for tangible and sustained growth.

Exercise 5: Visionary Letter to Your Future Self

(20 minutes)

In this imaginative exercise, write a heartfelt letter to your future self, visualizing a version of you who has overcome limiting beliefs and achieved remarkable growth. Pen down your aspirations and dreams for the person you aspire to become.

Describe the qualities, mindset, and achievements you envision for your future self. Be specific about the positive changes that you anticipate and intend to make to be the person you want to be. Share your hopes, triumphs, and the newfound beliefs that guide your journey. Take your time and be thorough with your inclusions.

Once you feel that you have incorporated everything into the letter seal it in an envelope labeled with the future date you've envisioned to become that person. Store it in a place where you can revisit it at that future date. If you are feeling brave share it with someone who you trust. They will act as your supporter as well as being able to hold you to its delivery. This exercise not only sets firm intentions for growth but creates a tangible, future-focused connection with your evolving self.

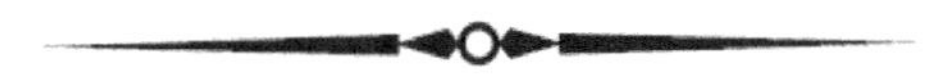

Conclusion

In this chapter, we have embarked on a journey to challenge negative beliefs and initiate a mindset transformation. We explored techniques like the visionary letter, dismantling barriers of negative self-talk, engaging in cognitive-behavioral exercises, and embracing gratitude practices and visualization. These practices serve to dismantle limiting beliefs and remove barriers that are currently hindering you from reaching your full potential.

As you continue this journey, remember that shifting limiting beliefs is a gradual process that requires patience, consistent effort, and the understanding that growth is an ongoing process. May the exercises provided, culminating in the visionary letter, serve as your ongoing companions, guiding you toward a mindset infused with positivity, resilience, and boundless growth as you stride toward your envisioned future self.

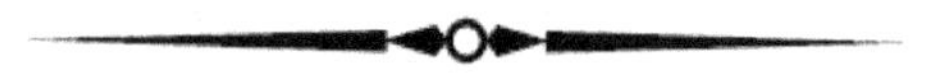

Chapter 6: Introducing the R.E.L.E.A.S.E. Framework

"The only person you are destined to become is the person you decide to be." [1]

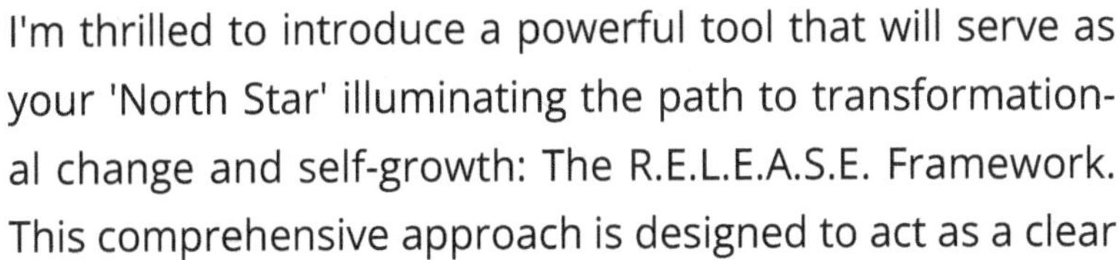

I'm thrilled to introduce a powerful tool that will serve as your 'North Star' illuminating the path to transformational change and self-growth: The R.E.L.E.A.S.E. Framework. This comprehensive approach is designed to act as a clear

---

1. Ralph Waldo Emerson (n.d.) As cited in James Jackson (2024) End Self-Sabotage and Stop Fighting with Yourself!

step-by-step guide to aid you through the process of shedding old patterns, embracing change, and evolving into the best version of yourself. Sounds great right?

So, let's examine this supportive framework and unlock the keys to your evolution.

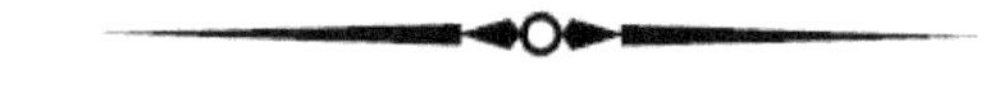

R.E.L.E.A.S.E. Overview

The R.E.L.E.A.S.E. Framework stands as a shining star, illuminating the path to self-transformation. Each letter represents a crucial step in this journey, collectively forming a detailed roadmap for your growth. Everyone loves a great analogy! Let's together break down the significance of each step of the process.

R - Reflect:

Reflection is the cornerstone of self-awareness and personal growth. In this step, we pause to look inward, examining our thoughts, emotions, and behaviors. It's a conscious effort to understand ourselves at a deeper level, unraveling the layers that have shaped our identity.

Reflection is a gentle exploration of our inner being achieved by engaging in practices like journaling, meditation, or introspective conversations. During this phase, we can reflect on our values, passions, and the beliefs that shape our reality. This lays the foundation for self-awareness, a crucial aspect of any transformative journey.

E - Embrace:

Embracing change is often easier said than done. Very few people actively seek out transformative change as it often lies outside of their comfort zone. This step invites us to acknowledge and accept the aspects of ourselves that may need a bit of transformation. It's about shedding our resistance and opening our arms to the positive possibilities that change can bring.

Embracing change requires a shift in mindset. Instead of resisting the unknown, we need to practice acceptance of it. We need to acknowledge areas for improvement, welcome new perspectives, and recognize that change is a constant and positive force in our lives.

L - Let Go:

Letting go is a liberating act. Here, we release the grip of past experiences, limiting beliefs, and self-imposed constraints. It's a courageous step that frees us from the shackles of our history, allowing space in our lives for new growth and exciting possibilities.

Letting go is akin to decluttering your emotional space. During this phase, we Identify and release attachments to past experiences, grudges, and self-limiting beliefs. This step is a profound act of self-compassion, creating room for our personal growth and renewal.

E - Evolve:

Evolution is the natural outcome of Reflect, Embrace, and Let Go. In this step, we actively engage in the process of personal development. It involves setting intentions, defining goals, and taking intentional steps toward the person we aspire to be.

By defining our aspirations, breaking them down into actionable tasks, and celebrating each milestone we achieve forward momentum that propels us toward our future intended self.

A - Align:

Alignment brings harmony to our journey. It's about aligning our actions, values, and goals. This step ensures that our transformation is not just surface-level but a holistic realignment of our internal compass.

This phase seeks to harmonize your actions to create your authentic self whilst removing internal stressors. This fosters a sense of completeness of purpose.

S - Seek Support:

Transformation doesn't happen in isolation. Seeking support is a vital step that involves reaching out to trusted individuals, mentors, or communities that can provide guidance, encouragement, and accountability. Together, we are stronger than when we are alone.

Seeking support is a courageous act, not a sign of weakness. Identifying individuals or communities that resonate with your journey is a strength. Engage in open and honest conversations, sharing your challenges and victories. The collective strength of a supportive network is immeasurable.

E - Empower:
Empowerment is the culmination of the R.E.L.E.A.S.E. journey. As we reflect, embrace, let go, evolve, align, and seek support, we empower ourselves to lead a life aligned with our truest desires and aspirations.

Through empowerment, you gain a realization of your inner strength and ultimate resilience. Celebrate your growth, acknowledge your capabilities, and embrace the lessons learned along the way. This step solidifies your newfound sense of self and purpose with action.

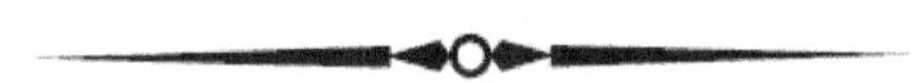

So why now?

If the R.E.L.E.A.S.E. framework is so good why wait until halfway through the book to introduce it? Well, that is a very good question. Often those who write self-help books develop a framework that serves to show the immensity of the journey ahead. Yes, it forms a clear path of progression but if that path is long and arduous many lose faith in reaching the destination. They often fall by the wayside early on and question why they ever started in the first place. This then reinforces their negative self-image. Not so you, my fine bibliophiles, yep you may need to look that one up. You are already well on your way to decoding your inner being and setting it on the path of transformation. You have already tackled a number of these framework elements in the chapters read and the exercises undertaken by following the more generic change methodology of awareness, acceptance, adoption, and advocacy. Whilst that process underpins this more detailed framework, we will now connect the two to drive your development forward at pace.

Let's take a detailed look at the stages and the core actions that you have already completed.

Reflect:

Reflect is all about gaining deep understanding and learnings from your past as well as your present to realize the full detriment that self-sabotaging has been having on your life. We have spent a lot of time from Chapter 1 onward, focusing on this point. From identifying outward signs such as procrastination, over-commitment, and staying within your comfort zone to the negative choices that you have made and the consequences of them. We also learned how those decisions impacted those around you causing a ripple effect of negative impact. In Chapter 2 you began to identify the triggers that lay behind those decisions and the emotions that were dragged alongside. We also crossed from waking days to sleeping opportunities using your dreams to identify and rehearse more positive approaches.

Embrace:

Within the embrace phase, which is about creating inner strength, shedding resistance to change, and understanding your current and future values and beliefs, we developed further understanding that led to cultivating self-compassion. This included journaling as well as mindful meditation practices from Chapter 3. In Chapter 4 we continued exploring past wounds to overcome and build inner resilience. You learned how to fortify yourself both physically and mentally, building strength for the journey ahead. We then ended the chapter by using affirmations to help heal with self-compassion, all designed to act as a support mechanism for change.

Let go:

In Chapter 5 we transitioned to letting go by identifying and challenging negative self-talk and our limiting beliefs. We also used Gratitude to focus on the positives in our lives which we could use to aid us in our motivation for change.

Evolve:

In Chapter 5 also we touched on Evolve as we moved from identifying and challenging to reframing our beliefs to form more positive outcomes. We also started to visualize our future selves and formed the intent and determination for change. We also momentarily slipped forward into Seeking

Support by exploring the opportunity that support groups hold for encouragement and accountability.

Conclusion

Wow! Just look how far you have come!

You are motoring along, heading down the highway of self-help in the blink of an eye. Ahead lies the combination of all of your great work and some further strategies, methods, tips, and ideas, along with the odd exercise or two. Now we will continue gaining development momentum as we travel onward at warp speed. Yes, Scotty, those engines can take it!

Together we will look deeper into applying the R.E.L.E.A .S.E. framework to our daily quest to end self-sabotage. We will also examine those hard-to-reach places with the accuracy of a Colgate Toothbrush. You know the ones I mean, where problems gather such as those troublesome relationships and those even more troublesome addictive behaviors. Together we will eliminate your self-destructive tendencies providing a fresh clean start to every day, all without the need for mouthwash.

Chapter 7: Application of the R.E.L.E.A.S.E. Framework

"The only limit to our realization of tomorrow will be our doubts of today." [1]

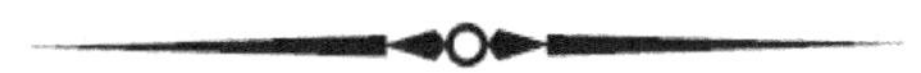

Now that the Dilithium crystals have all been warmed up we will speed ahead into the application phase of the

---

1. - Franklin D. Roosevelt(n.d.) As cited in James Jackson (2024) End Self-Sabotage and Stop Fighting with Yourself!

journey. The R.E.L.E.A.S.E. process is about to unfold in a more practical realm. Having traversed the realms of self-awareness, exploration, and understanding it is now time to put theory into practice, to wield the power of the R.E. and L. letters of our framework to shape the course of our interactions and behaviors. Sounds Exciting doesn't it?

Let's do it!

Practical Application of R.E.L.E.A.S.E. (Early Stage Recap)

In the early stages of applying the R.E.L.E.A.S.E. framework, our focus has been on setting the foundation for change. These hands-on exercises are designed to bridge the gap between self-awareness and proactive transformation. Let's recap the initial stages that are used to instigate practical shifts in your daily life. You will need your trusted and I suspect overflowing journal to hand.

Exercise 1: Reflect and Record

(30 minutes)

Begin by reflecting on the insights that you have gained throughout the R.E.L. phases so far. What behavioral patterns have you identified? What triggers have you found that initiated your self-sabotaging reactions? Record these observations as a summary on a dedicated page. Use headers such as **'Identified Patterns'** and **'Associated triggers'.** This consolidation serves to form a clear and concise roadmap for understanding your current behavioral landscape.

Next, if you have not already done so, identify specific scenarios or interactions where self-sabotage tends to surface most readily. What are the specific situations that cause these triggers to provoke a response? Be detailed and specific. This reflective process is the groundwork for creating targeted action plans. If you have already completed this task then transfer the main scenarios to the same page under a column headed **'Situations'**.

Exercise 2: Create Your Self-Sabotage Map

(30-60 minutes)

Use the newly summarized information to create a visual interpretation of your self-sabotage tendencies as a map with key destinations marked by triggers. Pinpoint the locations where self-sabotage often occurs. Are there specific environments, relationships, or situations that consistently lead to negative behaviors? By mapping these triggers, you will gain a spatial understanding of your challenges. It could look something like this: The event could be at work, the trigger may be critical responses, the emotions could be anger, frustration, self-hate, and fear of failure and the behavior could be defensiveness, stubbornness, and a lack of applied listening. This by the way could have been used to describe myself when I first started my career. I may have been studying Psychology but it didn't stop me from exhibiting these very same symptoms of self-destructive behavior. Thank god I took to reading my own books!

Now, create a legend for your map. List which emotional responses or actions accompany each trigger. Understanding the terrain of your self-sabotage landscape equips you with the knowledge needed for strategic intervention which we will later cover.

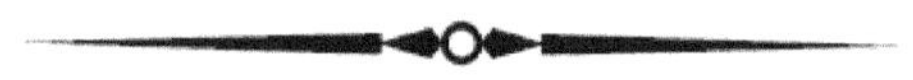

Creating Personalized Action Plans

With a clearer understanding of your self-sabotage landscape, it's time to craft personalized action plans. These plans will act as your guideposts, leading you away from self-sabotaging patterns and toward more constructive behaviors.

Activity 1: Defining Your Destination

(20-30 minutes)

You should already have identified the person you want to become and a timeline to complete that transformation using your letter to your future self. If not then please complete that exercise from Chapter 5 now. Envision what qualities, habits, and interactions characterize this ideal version of yourself. Be challenging to yourself. Don't wimp out with minor changes. This is your greatest opportunity to transform into the best version of yourself. So make it count. Define your destination clearly using highly descriptive words. This is the anchor for your action plans.

Activity 2: Break It Down

(30-60 minutes)

Breaking down your destination into manageable steps or waypoints is the next crucial step. Identify specific behaviors and responses that align with your desired future self. Your description to date is likely set at a more holistic level so take your time to really dig deep into each behavior change. You may have many to consider. Once you have clearly defined the first, then ask yourself which behaviors sit beneath it and keep repeating this until you have pinpointed the exact behavior and response that needs to change. For example, if your destination is improved communication, consider breaking it down into active listening, assertive expression, and empathetic understanding. You can always improve your active listening but if you don't also improve your empathy toward the person who you are listening to you may well miss the importance and nuance of the conversation. Once you have nailed the first behavior then go on to the next and so forth until you have a complete list of behaviors, sub-behaviors, and responses. These are your transformation actions.

Activity 3: The Micro-Habit Challenge

(10 minutes)

Embark on a micro-habit challenge. After reviewing your identified behavior and response changes select just one small, manageable behavior aligned with your destination and commit to practicing it consistently for a set period. Micro-habits are the building blocks for larger behavioral change. It is also a great way to start your transformation journey. OK so maybe it's a small step on the highway to success, but the first step is always the most important. Once complete you will be able to bask in the realization that change can happen and you can lead it.

Activity 4: Design Your Response Matrix

(ad-hoc)

Use your self-sabotage map to anticipate potential triggers. You now have recognized what they are and now we need to design a response matrix that outlines alternative reactions that you could take. It's like finding your way through a minefield. In the past, you would have blundered your way into and through it with scant regard for the explosions that you were setting off in your wake but now you have the secret route to negotiate them. If, for instance, criticism triggers negative self-talk, pre-plan responses that involve self-compassion and constructive reflection. If you find yourself heading down the hellish road to argument city with your loved one over something that you have done or not done take a moment to man or woman up and face the issue with a new focus. Perhaps your pre-planned response is to pause, consider, and reflect, knowing that this is the precise moment that you would normally capitulate to negative self-talk and get on the defensive. If that is through the criticism that you are hearing then your inner voice should be saying, "OK yep you are in the wrong but by accepting that you are not a failure, you are merely learning what to do better next time and your relationship will be better for it".

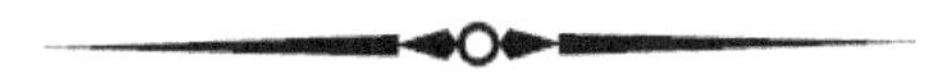

Tracking Progress and Milestones

As you implement your personalized action plans, tracking progress becomes paramount. Milestones are the markers of transformation, and acknowledging them fuels your motivation for continued growth. Here are a few options for you to consider:

Tracking Tool 1: Journaling Journey

Maintain transformation journal pages. Document daily experiences, and reflections, as you implement your action plans. The journal serves as a tangible record of your evolution, capturing both challenges and triumphs.

Tracking Tool 2: Milestone Celebrations

Celebrate the small victories. Completing your micro-habit challenge? Celebrate. Successfully redirecting a self-sabotaging response? Celebrate. These celebrations are not just acknowledgments; they are affirmations of your capability to effect change.

Tracking Tool 3: Accountability Partner

Consider engaging an accountability partner. Just to avoid misunderstanding and misery, that's not an 'Accountant'. The first will help you on your way forward, the second will mug you in a dark alley. Sorry to the countless accountants who are reading this book.

Find someone that you trust and share your goals and action plans with them. Arrange regular check-ins which will provide you with external support and insights, enhancing your commitment to the transformative journey. Once the cat's out of the bag then it's hard to get him back in without a lot of scratches.

Conclusion

So dear readers, just like the old classic Kill Bill this section comes in two parts but without all the shouting and samurai sword swishing about. We have just covered the 'R' for Reflect, the 'E' for Embrace, and the 'L' for Letting Go. Whilst we will shortly look into specific and more destructive behaviors over some of the following Chapters it is good to realize that you are already well on your way to successfully dealing with your self-sabotaging tendencies. You have already laid the most important groundwork for profound change. Something worth celebrating I feel.

The journey ahead is a dynamic process, and your commitment to these practical exercises propels you toward a future marked by intentional interactions and positive outcomes.

May your application of R.E.L.E.A.S.E. bring forth the transformative power you hold within or as a good friend of mine once said "May the force be with you" for the next stage of the journey.

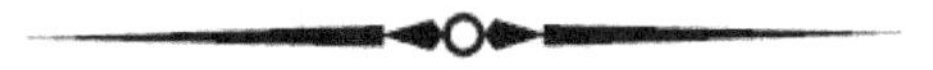

Chapter 8 Integrating R.E.L.E.A.S.E. into your Daily Routine

"Your life does not get better by chance, it gets better by change." [1]

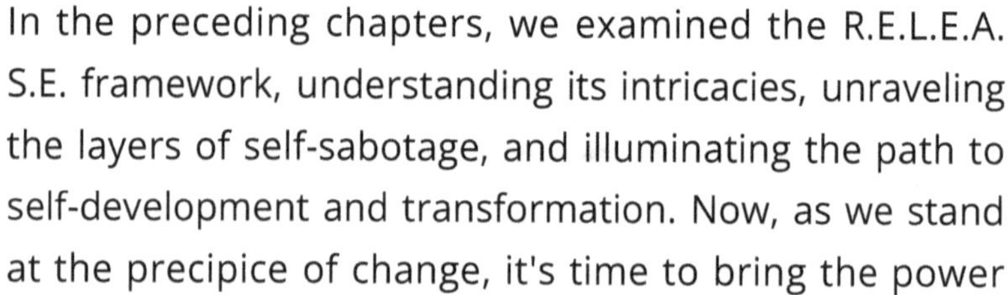

In the preceding chapters, we examined the R.E.L.E.A.
S.E. framework, understanding its intricacies, unraveling
the layers of self-sabotage, and illuminating the path to
self-development and transformation. Now, as we stand
at the precipice of change, it's time to bring the power

---

1. Jim Rohn(n.d.) As cited in James Jackson (2024) End
   Self-Sabotage and Stop Fighting with Yourself!

of R.E.L.E.A.S.E. into the rhythm of your daily life. In this chapter, we'll explore strategies, practical tools, and inter-active activities to seamlessly integrate the framework into your routine, fostering long-term resilience and growth. Consider it a bit like brushing your teeth in the morning, both will make you smile but only one will give you that minty freshness all day long.

Daily Integration for Long-term Resilience

Strategies for Seamless Adoption:

The key to lasting change lies in the integration of new practices into your daily routine. To make R.E.L.E.A.S.E. a part of your life, consider the following strategies over and above what has been discussed so far: Consistency is the key here along with a total focus on changing your approach to destructive influences.

1. **Morning Reflections:** Start your day with a few moments of mindful reflection. Review your R.E .L.E.A.S.E. goals, affirmations, and the action plan that you've crafted. Also, review your latest journal entries to relive the moments and emotions that you experienced at the time of your entries. Use all of these inputs to visualize success and set a positive tone for the day ahead.

2. **Mindful Moments:** Infuse mindfulness into your routine. Whether during your commute, a coffee break, or a quiet moment at home, practice mindful breathing. This simple yet powerful exercise grounds you in the present, fostering resilience.

3. **Daily Affirmation Ritual:** Repeat your collected personalized affirmations daily. Embed them in your morning routine or tie them to specific activities like brushing your teeth. Affirmations, like daily mantras, serve as reminders of your growth journey.

4. **Scheduled Check-ins:** Set aside time each day for a brief check-in with yourself. Reflect on your experiences, challenges, and victories. Adjust your mindset if needed and celebrate all the small wins as well as the bigger ones. Consistent reflection is a cornerstone of the R.E.L.E.A.S.E. process.

5. **Integrated Learning:** Weave the principles of R.E.L.E.A.S.E. into your knowledge acquisition. Listen to podcasts, read articles, or engage in discussions related to self-growth and resilience. This continuous learning reinforces the framework's principles and provides you with valuable additional insights.

Techniques for Sustained Adoption

Sustaining adoption requires a thoughtful approach. Consider these techniques to keep R.E.L.E.A.S.E. alive in your daily routine:

1. **Progress Journaling:** Maintain a progress journal. OK, just how many journals can one person own? I know, I know... We could spend our whole day just writing things down and never getting to do anything with them, or indeed anything at all except drive up the price of journals. This is just one approach to consider. Regularly documenting your experiences, insights, and the evolution of your mindset means that you not only have to recall and remember those positive moments to write them down but you can later bask in the warmth of re-living them when you read them back. This creates a virtuous circle of positive reinforcement

2. **Accountability Partnerships:** I mentioned this briefly before but getting someone onboard and on your side will really help. A problem shared is a problem halved. Share your R.E.L.E.A.S.E. journey with a trusted friend or family member and then you can establish a system of mutual accountability. Discuss challenges, share achievements, and offer support when needed. Great if they are on their own journey too because you can reciprocate the support.

3. **Adaptability in Practice:** Life is dynamic, and so should be your approach to R.E.L.E.A.S.E. Be adaptable in integrating the framework into your changing circumstances. Flexibility ensures that it remains a relevant and effective tool and you don't get weighed down by the bureaucratic practice of strict timings and actions. Now I am certainly not saying to you to abandon all reason and ignore what has been writen, but I am saying that we are all wonderfully different, with different circumstances, different pressures, and quite frankly different lives. There is no such thing as one size fits all unless you live on a catwalk. We must cut our own cloth to the world we live in and make sure that we keep moving forward no matter what circumstances pan out. Basically, be intentionally kind to yourself just as much as you are being strict to ensure a happy balance. But never let it slide.

4. **Rewards System:** Introduce a rewards system tied to your R.E.L.E.A.S.E. goals. I love rewards! I use this tool with myself all the time, even now as I am typing away. Do you know that I am only able to grab a nice cuppa with a chocolate biscuit when I've finished this entire Chapter? Now that's being a tough taskmaster! And I can't even blame someone else. So celebrate each milestone with small, meaningful rewards. This will further serve as positive reinforcement which will enhance your motivation and reinforce the habit loop.

5. **Holistic Lifestyle Alignment:** Align other aspects of your lifestyle with the R.E.L.E.A.S.E. framework. This will also make a huge difference. Try exploring complementary practices like yoga, meditation, or hobbies that promote holistic well-being and reinforce positive habits. Try extending this outside your comfort zone. If you are lacking in a little self-confidence then getting involved in team sports may help. If you seldom schedule any moments to just be yourself from a hectic home life, then determine to carve out a specific instance just for you. Don't take any arguments from anyone else, just do it. Take a walk, relax in a spa, or simply lock the door and read a great book – like this one :)

Ongoing Support and Interactive Activities

Embarking on a self-transformation journey can be both empowering and challenging. Whilst reading a book on the subject will help and engaging in the exercises and activities suggested will help even more, it's good to seek additional support where it exists. To provide such ongoing support, consider the following guidance and suggestions:

1. **Virtual Support Groups:** Connect with like-minded individuals through virtual support groups or

forums. Share your R.E.L.E.A.S.E. experiences, gain insights from others, and build a community that bolsters your resilience. I understand that this may sound a bit traditional or you may balk at the fact of seeking a group of other self-sabotaging sufferers but there is a good reason why this is being suggested. Think of Alcoholics Anonymous which is the go-to example. They have this nailed down tight. They realize that just telling people how bad it is to drink a lot and sticking a leaflet in their hands, would not get very far. But sharing each other's life experiences and offering shared comfort and support works far better. It is more relatable and real. So virtual, or better still, real support groups can help your continued transformation away from self-sabotaging tendencies even when times are tough.

2. **Bi-weekly Reflection Prompts:** Receive bi-weekly reflection prompts via email or a dedicated app. These prompts encourage deeper introspection, helping you navigate specific aspects of the R.E.L .E.A.S.E. framework. Simply set them up on a smart home assistant as a scheduled reminder.

3. **Interactive Webinars:** Participate in interactive webinars led by experts in self-growth. These sessions can offer additional tools, insights, and opportunities for Q&A, fostering a sense of community and shared learning.

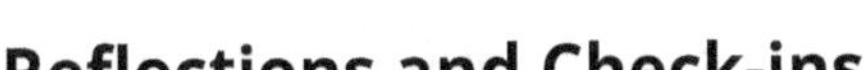

Reflections and Check-ins

Regular reflection and check-ins are great tools for maintaining your momentum. Here are a few suggestions that you can incorporate into your more medium-term routine planning:

1. **Monthly Progress Reports:** Set aside time at the end of each month to create a comprehensive progress report. Reflect on the highs and lows, reassess your goals, and acknowledge the growth you've experienced as well as the challenges you have faced.

2. **Goal Adjustment Sessions:** Life evolves, and so do your goals. Conduct quarterly goal adjustment sessions. Assess whether your objectives still align with your current aspirations and make adjustments accordingly. Remember there are no hard and fast rules here. The overriding objective is to maintain your momentum and progression toward a successful life without any self-destructive elements.

3. **360-Degree Feedback:** Now if you have engaged others close to you in your mission to overcome your sabotaging habit then a 360-degree feedback

session could be something to consider. If that person is your partner or even a really good friend then the feedback will likely be more complete and honest. At the same time involving these people could mean being quite brave and accepting their feedback with grace and in the spirit it is given in. Ultimately trusted individuals who are already supporting you will make this exercise highly beneficial. You will need to seek open and honest feedback covering multiple facets of your life—personal, professional, and social. A 360-degree perspective offers a holistic view of your growth, highlighting areas for further development opportunities.

4. **Celebration Rituals:** Design celebration rituals for more significant milestones. Whether it's a special dinner, a weekend getaway, or a symbolic gesture, these rituals mark your achievements and reinforce the positive changes that you are making. This is all about being kind to yourself, recognizing the progress you are making, and reinforcing the benefits of staying the course.

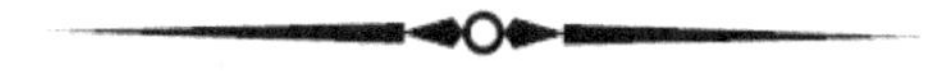

Conclusion

As you integrate R.E.L.E.A.S.E. into your daily routine, remember that resilience is not a destination but a continuous evolution. Embrace the ebb and flow of the process and your progress. Celebrate your victories, and learn from challenges. Whilst the above is intentionally very generic and can be applied to many conditions that affect or impact our lives they are nonetheless extremely powerful reinforcements for you to use.

The R.E.L.E.A.S.E. framework is your sundial, guiding you toward a life infused with warmth and positivity, resilience, and boundless growth. Through these daily, weekly, monthly, and quarterly practices, coupled with ongoing support, you are not just adopting a framework; you are crafting a resilient and empowered version of yourself—one intentional day at a time.

And now for that Cup of tea....

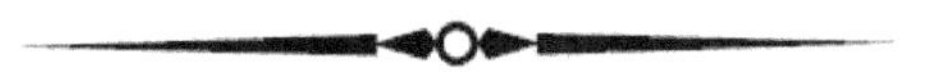

Chapter 9: Overcoming Relationship Challenges

"Ultimately the bond of all companionship, whether in marriage or in friendship, is conversation."[1]

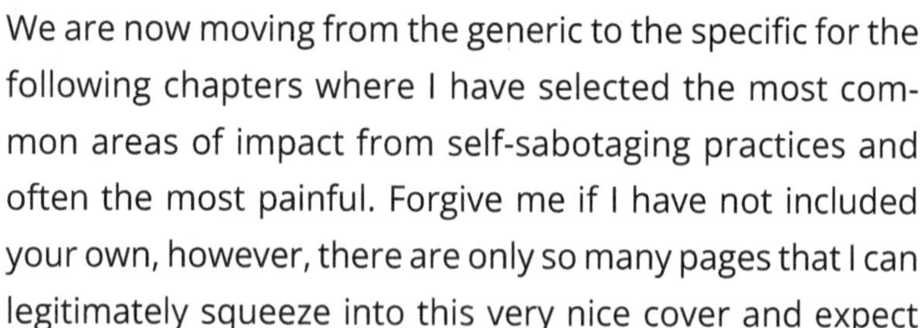

We are now moving from the generic to the specific for the following chapters where I have selected the most common areas of impact from self-sabotaging practices and often the most painful. Forgive me if I have not included your own, however, there are only so many pages that I can legitimately squeeze into this very nice cover and expect

---

1. Oscar Wilde, 1905, "De Profundis"

you all to read. The process of overcoming any situations of destructive impact, including those outside the ones of focus remains the same, so you have not missed out and may at the same time find some fascinating reading to reflect upon. Sometimes as we compare what we read to our situations we realize the inescapable truth that our behavior overspills into many areas of our lives and that of those around us.

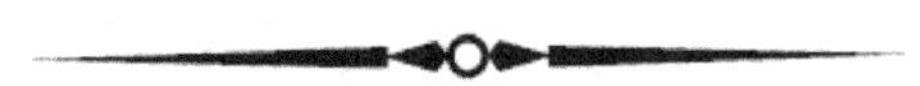

Relationships

Relationships can be tough at the best of times. Whether you are young and just starting out on them or old and still wrestling with them, they are arguably one of the most important aspects of our brief lives. Relationships exist between lovers, mothers, fathers, sons and daughters, teammates, workmates, and even drinking buddies. They are intricate, sometimes delicate, make us laugh and cry, send our hearts soaring, or plunge us to the depths of despair. Some of us dive into them, some of us avoid them like the plague but for many relationships happen, flourish, deepen, and become long-term. They support our perception of our self-worth and provide purpose and meaning to our lives through shared experiences and emotional attachment. However, when self-sabotage enters the picture, these relationships can fracture, putting a strain on the very foundation of our connections. In this chapter, we'll delve into the complexities of relationship dynamics affected by self-sabotage, explore the psychological impacts, examine practical tools for healing, and draw inspiration from real-life narratives of individuals who successfully navigated through these challenges.

We will also use this delicate topic to actively utilize the R.E.L.E.A.S.E. process. Think of this as a test case for the process, a show-and-tell session. We will use our current knowledge of the process to proceed to address the relationship challenges that are a result of self-sabotage.

Let us progress step-by-step.

Understanding Relationship Dynamics Affected by Self-Sabotage

The Roots of Self-Sabotage:
Deep-seated fears, insecurities, or limiting beliefs often serve as the breeding ground for self-sabotage within relationships. These tendencies, from a psychological perspective, can often be traced back to earlier life experiences, which shape our attachment style and influence our ap-

proach to intimacy, connection, and even collaboration in professional settings.

"Your task is not to seek for love, but merely to seek and find all the barriers within yourself that you have built against it."
- Rumi

Acknowledging the Impact:

Imagine a scenario where the fear of vulnerability leads to overwhelming trust issues resulting in the constant questioning of a partner's love. Or when that same fear asserts itself in a reluctance to take risks and hinders collaborative efforts in a more professional environment. How about focusing on a more social setting with friends where a fear of vulnerability could threaten the free sharing of stories and experiences placing you on the periphery of the group? These self-sabotaging beliefs, when left unchecked, create emotional distance, misunderstandings, and conflicts, affecting the very fabric of our relationships. Remember that these examples are all born from a single underlying emotive driver. There can be many such drivers, underlying insecurities, or limiting beliefs that we have constructed over time. Each can give rise to negative thinking and cases of self-sabotage which can destroy relationships, hinder career advancement, and worse still, initiate a repeating pattern of behavior that becomes habit-forming. The good news is that you are actively pursuing ways to break this destructive cycle when many don't even realize that they are in one.

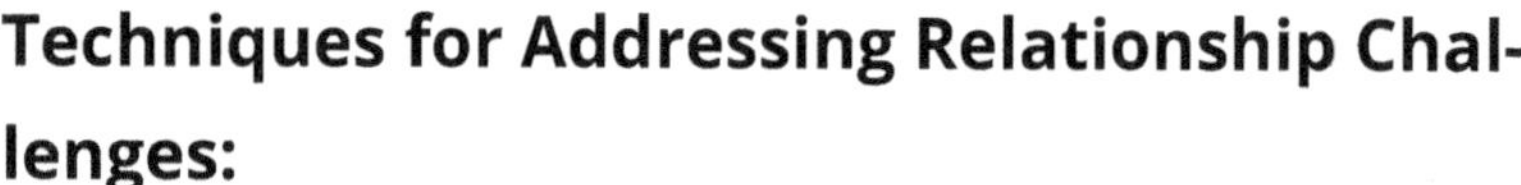

Techniques for Addressing Relationship Challenges:

Now assuming that you have used the practices already described you would have realized just how broadly your self-destructive tendencies impact your life. Remember that awareness is the critical starting point for any method to address such tendencies. Without awareness and then acceptance that the fault doesn't lie with others but with yourself, you can't hope to move forward. It's a bit like trying to convince someone that rice cakes are a tasty snack if they want to lose weight and that a dozen chicken wings is probably inversely not. I mean have you tried a rice cake...But seriously if you have no overwhelming desire to lose weight, even if you know you should, then there is no way in the world you would tackle a dried-out old piece of cardboard. You need to fully accept that you need to change and not simply play lip service to the idea.

So let's consider the scenario that you are not only aware there is a problem but by following the R.E.L.E.A.S.E . process you have also accepted that you are responsible for that problem. These two stages are representative of the R of reflect, and the E of Embrace. What do you do next? Well, you need to consider what to do to change things right? This could be described as adoption. Adoption of actions that can be used to address the issue and work toward repairing the situation which in this case is a relationship. Adoption can include the L for Letting go, the E for Evolve as that is the culmination of your actions in the earlier phases of the process, and the A of Align which we will come to shortly. Hopefully, now you can see how each phase of the process connects to enable you to move forward step-by-step. This in turn provides momentum. Consider it a sabotage solution Lego set because... well everyone loves Lego right?

Below are three exercises that can be used consecutively to address awareness, acceptance, and adoption. The first of these exercises you should already be familiar with as we have already introduced it earlier. However, for those of you who, naughty, naughty, may have skimmed a bit then I have included it here as a reminder. For all of those goody-two-shoes who have already used it, I love you all, and you can skip on to exercise two.

1. Self-Reflection: Navigating the Depths of Your Psyche

Embarking on a voyage of self-reflection is akin to donning a skin-tight scuba suit for an exploration into the depths of your psyche. I encourage you all to not merely doggy-paddle upon the surface but to plunge headlong into the ocean of your past experiences and the associated attachment patterns that have formed. This psychological reflective deep-dive will unveil the intricate coral formations of your relational history, revealing the roots of self-sabotage that have taken hold. By taking the time to intentionally look back into your life at those critical moments that impacted your thinking and emotional responses to relationship forming, you can decipher the root causes. When you undertake this task make sure that you have time set aside in a quiet space with no distractions. Please also circle back to explore chapters from one to four if you are not certain of what to do here as I will intentionally not be going into detail. Needless to say, you need to use the numerous exercises listed to excavate the key learnings from your emotional history by searching within yourself and pinpointing the historical impact points that have influenced your thinking. These could be earlier relationship trauma, pressure, abuse, or incidents that scarred your being.

This core undertaking of self-reflection acts as a lens through which you can observe your emotional ecosystem, recognizing certain patterns and uncovering your submerged beliefs. By doing so, you will unearth the fertile ground for meaningful change. This psychological archaeology is also a versatile tool, equally applicable to personal, professional, and social spheres. Yes, here one size does fit all. The self-awareness forged through this process becomes your catalyst for intentional transformative growth. You not only become aware of the problem and its core root causes but also understand its severity through introspection and the exercises described. You are enabled to move on to acceptance through this same introspection. Acceptance that things need to change

"In the depth of winter, I finally learned that within me there lay an invincible summer." - Albert Camus

2. Open Communication: Building Bridges to Deeper Connections

So to the next stage, having become aware and accepting that changes are needed.

Picture yourself as the architect of your emotional landscape, equipped with detailed blueprints for crafting bridges that connect you to those around you. In the realm of relationships, these bridges are not mere physical structures but conduits for emotions, thoughts, and understanding. Open communication is your master plan, your guide to constructing these vital connections.

Open communication can be a scary thought. Few like to open up to lovers, friends, and colleagues as they can feel vulnerable. However, we need to learn that it is that very vulnerability that is our strength when honestly expressed in building or rebuilding relationships. Envision what it would feel like to repair all of your damaged relationships.

Let's take a moment to understand the reason for open communication, its benefits, and how best to use it.

The Blueprint:

Much like the architect who envisions a building's grand design, you're tasked with envisioning the structure of your relationships. Open communication becomes your best way to create a solid blueprint, laying the foundation for securing improved emotional attachments going forward. Think of it as the sturdy groundwork upon which you'll construct the bridges that connect you with others around you. I also view open dialogue as a craft knife cutting through all of the crap that builds up between individuals. Often it is a personal and heartfelt discussion without accusation and emboldened with acceptance and ownership that enables a positive movement to begin.

Navigating Stormy Seas:

Relationships, much like the weather, can be highly unpredictable. Open communication doesn't just celebrate the sunny days of joy and laughter; it also equips you to navigate the stormy seas of fears, and concerns. Being the architect of your emotional connections means expressing the full spectrum of your experiences. It's about sharing not only the joys but also the vulnerabilities that make us human. It's about being honest and above all authentic.

The Mortar of Vulnerability:

Now getting back to the subject of feeling vulnerable, imagine your vulnerability as the mortar that binds the bricks of understanding and empathy together. This mortar is not a weakness but a true strength, holding your emotional connections securely together. It's the honesty that makes your emotional bridges resilient and capable of withstanding the tests of time. As you express your true self, your emotional connections will also become authentic and profound.

Countering Self-Sabotage:

Now you know that at some point self-sabotage will attempt to raise its ugly head. In your relationship design it is often self-sabotage who has acted as an unforeseen disruptor. Open communication with those whom you want better relationships with will become the counterforce to this menace. By expressing your emotions authentically, you are diluting the opportunity and potency of self-sabotaging tendencies. It's the act of laying bare your emotional state that makes it harder for self-sabotage to find fertile ground.

Constructing Sturdy Bridges:

As you articulate your emotional landscapes to partners, colleagues, or friends, you're not merely sharing words; you're constructing sturdy bridges built through shared understanding and emotional reciprocity. This means that you can avoid misunderstandings and strengthen emotional bonds. In personal relationships, these conduits foster intimacy and deeper connection. In professional collaborations, they facilitate teamwork, mutual trust, and respect. In your social circle, they create bonds that can last a lifetime.

Conduits for Shared Understanding:

Through your renewed actions built from awareness and acceptance, you are actively adopting practices to repair damaged relationships. Yes, you need to put in the hard graft here as it is likely that your newly unearthed self-sabotaging root causes are the reason why the relationships are strained in the first place. By expressing your feelings openly, you're inviting others to do the same and at the same time creating a platform for shared understanding and appreciation. The exchange of thoughts and emotions forms the basis of deep connections. In personal, professional, and social spheres, these conduits become the lifelines of relationships encouraging reciprocity.

In essence, open communication is your toolkit for becoming the master architect of your relationships. It's not about perfection but about the art of construction, allowing you to build bridges that withstand the complexities of human connection and counteract the disruptive forces of self-sabotage. As you craft these emotional conduits, you're not just communicating; you're creating a masterpiece of connection that enriches every facet of your life.

"Communication is the solvent of all problems, therefore, communication skills are the foundation for personal development." - Peter Shepherd

3. Setting Boundaries: Forging Your Psychological Armor

In the realm of psychology, setting boundaries is similar to adopting the role of a blacksmith forging a suit of armor to act as a shield around your self-concept. Take a moment to envision that armor and shield as a metaphysical force field, a dynamic boundary that surrounds you defining the contours of your personal space and autonomy. You are not merely an observer of this phenomenon but the artisan in the workshop creating your psychological defenses. In short, these barriers of protection and defense are created by yourself and help to align your inner being to the situations that may arise from new or existing relationships.

Crafting Your Psychological Armor:

In the act of crafting such armor, you are molding the boundaries that will safeguard your psychological well-being. These boundaries are not rigid walls but dynamic shields, adapting to different scenarios in personal, professional, and social spheres. The act of crafting this psychological armor can be an empowering journey, allowing you to declare your commitment to maintaining security in every facet of your life. However in certain circumstances especially when you have encountered past trauma, these defenses can become overly exaggerated, acting as high walls excluding the possibility of emotional connection with others. In the act of becoming self-aware of past circumstances that have negatively informed your decision-making you also gain the power to reassess such defenses. The realization that these barriers are not set in stone empowers you to re-establish more person-appropriate self-defense measures which enable the reformation of emotional connections.

Appropriate Boundary Setting:

As mentioned forging your more appropriate levels of psychological armor is an empowering experience that allows you to establish boundaries, which can act as sentinels against the encroachment of self-sabotaging behaviors. These sentinels stand guard, ensuring that your inner sanctum remains untarnished by destructive tendencies. Recognize that the setting of appropriate boundaries can be an act of self-love and self-preservation without the need for the full exclusion of others or a barrier to forming valuable relationships. This practice forms a correctly weighted commitment to your mental and emotional well-being demarcating the line between healthy interdependence and enmeshment.

Following this process will allow you to craft a healthy environment that allows for meaningful connections without sacrificing your individual identity. By conducting this internal realignment and setting clear boundaries, you create an environment where relationships can flourish without being overshadowed by self-sabotage.

Parameters for Professional Collaboration:

In the professional landscape, your recalibrated psychological armor establishes parameters for collaboration without compromising individual identity. You can navigate the complex terrain of the workplace with confidence, knowing that your boundaries safeguard your autonomy while simultaneously fostering effective teamwork. It's a delicate balance of collaboration without surrender.

Nourishing Connections in Social Circles:

In social circles, your psychological armor ensures that connections are nourishing rather than depleting. By defining your personal space, you invite relationships that uplift and support you. Setting boundaries is not an act of exclusion; it's a conscious choice to surround yourself with the connections that contribute positively to your life whilst excluding those that don't.

Harmonious Bonds in Intimate Relationships:

Within the intimacy of romantic relationships, your psychological armor serves as the guardian of shared vulnerabilities and individual sanctuaries. It is a place to delicately craft a space where love and autonomy coexist. Setting boundaries becomes an artistry of alignment and connection, a carefully constructed balance between intimacy and self-preservation. These boundaries are not barriers but affirmations of individual identity within the shared space of love where you honor the sanctity of personal space while embracing the closeness that defines romantic connection. This delicate balance allows both partners to thrive as unique individuals while being deeply intertwined in the dance of love.

Within the cocoon of intimate connection, your boundaries become a compass for navigating emotional terrain.

They facilitate open communication about personal needs, desires, and fears, fostering a fulfilling relationship where both partners feel seen and understood. As you articulate your emotional landscapes, the boundaries you set become the framework for a resilient and thriving bond creating a space where both partners can express their true selves without fear of judgment. This conscious choice to define personal space within a deeply loving relationship is immensely empowering and transforms boundaries from limitations to open opportunities to create a beautiful and enduring connection.

A Guiding Quote:

"Your personal boundaries protect the inner core of your identity and your right to choices." - Gerard Manley Hopkins

Reader Narratives and Relationship Transformations

So in the previous sections, we have moved from the R.E.L.E. of Reflect, Embrace, Letting go, and Evolve, to include A for alignment and the E for Empowerment. Let's now examine some real-life examples where this step-by-step process has been successful at repairing relationships.

John and Sarah: Rebuilding Trust

John and Sarah's narrative unfolds as a psychological exploration of attachment dynamics. John's fear of abandonment, rooted in his earliest experiences from being in foster care, led to constant questioning. Deep down John's insecurities meant that he could never truly believe that in later life he had found a loving relationship with Sarah. This manifested itself in distrust, controlling behavior, and bouts of depression which ultimately negatively impacted his relationship as it had done in past relationships. Not only had this previously happened but because it was a repeating cycle it just reinforced John's limiting beliefs of his unworthiness to hold down long-term relationships as well as influencing his expectations of how lovers behave.

Through open communication and psychological insights gained in therapy, John and Sarah worked on rebuilding their trust in one another. Johns's journey through awareness and acceptance of his limiting beliefs enabled him to take a step back and manage his insecurities. During the process of using open and genuine dialogue, Sarah gained a profound understanding of his struggles and the resulting behaviors that John had exhibited in their relationship. Today, they can celebrate a resilient relationship, illustrating the transformative power of psychological awareness and open communication.

Inaya's Workplace Success

Inaya's fear of success, a psychological barrier rooted in her self-concept, hindered her professional growth. By recognizing this fact and undertaking periods of introspection Inaya realized that her earliest perceptions of abandonment by highly successful professional parents had shaped her own relationship beliefs. Being a young mother her fears of repeating this behavior with her child had negatively impacted her career. By letting go of this self-sabotaging belief and seeking mentorship she was able to confront these psychological barriers. Inaya's newfound proactive approach not only enabled her advancement but also inspired positive changes in her work relationships, underscoring the profound impact of psychological insight.

Inaya's journey toward workplace success unveils the transformative power of the R.E.L.E.A.S.E. process. Recognizing her fear of success as a self-sabotaging tendency deeply rooted in her self-concept, Inaya embarked on a journey of self-discovery and growth.

Aaron's Social Liberation with R.E.L.E.A.S.E.

Aaron's charismatic yet self-sabotaging nature in social circles found liberation through the strategic deployment of the R.E.L.E.A.S.E. process. By undertaking reflection exercises Aaron understood that his fear of not being in control of situations led him to adopt an overly dominant and opinionated character in any social setting. Aaron established that as a child growing up in a hostile environment, his honed survival skills had included taking on a tough and determined persona that was incapable of being wrong under any circumstances. This strength of will had been appropriate to the environment that he had witnessed as a child but was wholly out of step with his adulthood. By re-evaluating his boundary setting and the psychological armor that shielded him from the encroachment of self-sabotaging behaviors Aarron was able to let go of these beliefs whilst realigning his inner self to enable relationship growth without fear of being vulnerable. This empowered him to participate far more openly in social gatherings without the need to take center stage and dominate discussions.

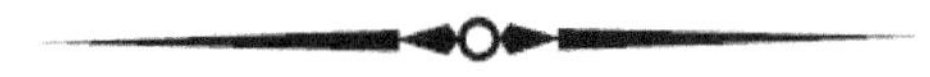

Conclusion

In the world of human connections, understanding the psychological underpinnings of self-sabotage is pivotal. Armed with psychological insights, effective tools, and wisdom drawn from real-life transformations across personal, professional, and social domains, you should now be able to see how the process can be used to counter self-sabotaging tendencies in relationship settings.

Chapter 10: Navigating the Work Environment

"It is impossible to live without failing at something unless you live so cautiously that you might as well not have lived at all, in which case you have failed by default." [1]

The Workplace

The average person will spend 90,000 hours at work over their lifetime, most of it awake. That is a scary figure. If we are spending a third of our lives at work and a third of our lives sleeping then it's probable that we see more of our work colleagues than anyone else in our lives. So if you

1.

are having negative relationships with them then that's a whole chunk of time spent being miserable. Now I have worked for some great businesses and for some utterly crap ones too. Whether you're thriving or surviving in this environment, one thing remains constant: people around you matter. If you hate each other's guts then irrespective of the quality of the business that you are in, you are simply not going to be enjoying a third of your life and that is a very sad thing indeed.

Now imagine if some of those 'hate your guts' relationships were actually down to you. Imagine if they all were. How bad would you feel? Not only are you hating a third of your life but you are inviting numerous co-workers to hate a third of theirs too. And remember this animosity rubs off onto the rest of your life too. Consider how many times you have returned home after a bad day at work and moaned to your partner just how bad everyone is and that your job utterly sucks!. So now a good percentage of the time you are spending with others is tarnished by your feelings of anger, frustration, and annoyance at the poor work rela- tionships that you may have been responsible for in the first place. Life can be kind of shit, can't it?

And if you hate where you work and the people you work with you are equally likely to lack the motivation to suc- ceed in the job that you are doing. Your professional view being so tarnished will lead to underperformance and a diminished likelihood of career advancement. So you may be stuck with those people you hate the guts of for a very long time.

But, hold on, there's a far more sunnier take on the situation; if you have resigned yourself to spending a third of your life hating work and everyone there and another ten percent or more moaning about it, then why not invest a small amount of time and energy understanding why the relationships are fractured and put them back together. The upside is that nearly half your life will be happy again. That would be a bit of a win, wouldn't it?

To make it a whole lot easier you have the solution here in your hands, or on your phone, kindle, or laptop, delete whichever is not applicable. The R.E.L.E.A.S.E. process can be applied here as well. Reflect on the situation, dig into your feelings, explore the emotional triggers, uncover your limiting beliefs, and dissect the moments that pushed you from positivity to negativity. Identify self-sabotaging instances, the triggers, and the associated emotions. Acknowledge the impacts of these episodes on both your personal and professional life, and envision how your life and career could have been different if you had responded differently. Wow, all that in just three sentences... Now let's see where all this takes us.

Managing Self-Sabotage at Work:

So you have undertaken all the actions previously described. You now understand which situations have been made worse by your self-sabotaging tendencies and the emotional drivers that have led to the responses and the behaviors that you have exhibited. If you simply held onto that knowledge and the enlightenment of realization then you would feel pretty sad with yourself. You now need to determine what you will do with that knowledge and how you will use your learnings to change those negative outcomes. Know too that it is very rare for anything to be irreparable. That goes equally for relationships as it does for career development. Where there is a will there is normally a way.

Now the time has come to put the rest of the process into action. Align, Seek Support, and Empowerment. Let's now have a look at some techniques that you can use for exactly that. Intentionally I have also included two exercises that you should be aware of from earlier as they are also critical here.

Emotional Check-Ins:

Embarking on a journey of self-awareness within the confines of your work environment requires regular emotional check-ins. Consider these moments as dedicated pauses in the hustle and bustle of your day, allowing you to reflect on your mental state. Begin by acknowledging your emotions, whether positive or negative, and discern any patterns that emerge. Are certain situations triggering negativity or self-sabotaging thoughts? By recognizing these patterns, you empower yourself to intervene and redirect your mindset.

Delve deeper into your emotional landscape during these check-ins. Uncover the root causes of negative emotions and self-sabotage. Are they linked to specific tasks, colleagues, or deadlines? You are likely to have these causes already detailed from earlier in your journal. Identifying the exact triggers provides a roadmap for targeted intervention. It could be an overwhelming workload, strained relationships, or the fear of failure. Armed with this understanding, you can take a breath and proactively address these issues, whether through personal strategies or collaborative efforts.

As you progress, actively work on shifting your mindset by introducing positive affirmations or visualization techniques to counteract negative thoughts. Embrace moments of gratitude and celebration, acknowledging your achievements, no matter how small. The goal is to cultivate a resilient and adaptable mindset that can navigate the challenges found in the work environment.

Constructive Communication:

Effective communication is the bedrock of a healthy work environment as discussed earlier. Engaging in open and constructive communication with colleagues transforms the workplace into a space where conflicts are addressed directly, fostering resolutions and a sense of unity. Here's how to navigate this, sometimes scary area, with newfound confidence and skill :

- **Initiate Conversations:** Don't shy away from initiating conversations, especially when you sense tension or conflicts. You may already know that you are the cause of the conflict or already suspect it. All you need is courage to rewrite the situation and the outcome. Addressing issues promptly prevents them from festering and escalating so don't procrastinate.

- **Active Listening:** Cultivate the art of active listening. Pay attention to your colleagues' perspectives without immediately formulating responses. This demonstrates respect and promotes a more collaborative atmosphere. Remember that active listening goes beyond just hearing the words and pretending that you are interested. You really do need to be interested as well as take note of the subtle cues, inclusions, and tonality. A person can say that everything is fine when you know damn well it isn't. Use your eyes to notice body language as well as spoken language as that is often a prime giveaway of how people are feeling, including yourself.

- **Use "I" Statements:** When expressing concerns or disagreements, frame them using "I" statements. This approach emphasizes personal experiences and feelings, reducing the likelihood of defensive reactions. Be understanding and empathetic to responses and talk from the heart. Be open for feedback even if you don't like what you hear and don't be defensive. Avoid the word 'but', such as "I agree with you, but". That means you don't agree at all. Let's not sugarcoat it.

- **Seek Solutions:** Focus on finding solutions rather than dwelling on problems. The past is the past, you are interested in seeking solutions for the current and future. Encourage a problem-solving mindset among your colleagues, emphasizing collective goals and mutual success. Be respectful and try not to rush responses without due thought. Loose talk costs lives. Seek mutual agreement and double-check that everyone is being honest when they agree to the resolution.

- **Regular Check-Ins:** Establish a culture of regular check-ins or feedback sessions. These can be informal discussions or more structured meetings, providing opportunities for open communication and continuous improvement. It also means that you are addressing any outstanding issues even if you didn't even know that one existed.

By actively engaging in constructive communication, you contribute to breaking down communication barriers, fostering trust, and creating a healthier work environment.

Team Building Activities:

Team-building activities extend beyond mere corporate rituals; they are potent tools for fortifying interpersonal relationships within the workplace. These activities serve as a bridge, connecting individuals on a more personal level and fostering camaraderie. Consider the following strategies to make these activities effective:

- **Diverse Experiences:** Select team-building activities that offer diverse experiences, catering to different interests and preferences. This ensures that everyone can actively participate, contribute and learn.

- **Inclusivity:** Ensure inclusivity in the choice of activities, considering the varied strengths and abilities of team members. This prevents the unintentional exclusion of certain individuals and promotes a sense of unity.

- **Reflect on Work Dynamics:** Tailor team-building activities to reflect and address specific work dynamics or challenges. This targeted approach can contribute to breaking down walls and enhancing collaboration.

- **Rotate Leadership Roles:** Introduce an element of shared leadership during team-building activities. Rotating leadership roles empowers team members to showcase their strengths and foster a collaborative spirit.

- **Encourage Open Reflection:** After each activity, encourage open reflection and discussion. This allows team members to share their experiences, insights, and takeaways, deepening their connections.

Team-building activities, when thoughtfully chosen and executed, have the potential to dismantle the barriers contributing to self-sabotage. They foster a sense of community and shared purpose, creating an environment where individuals are more likely to support and uplift one another. This 'one team' togetherness will extend beyond the immediate and help strengthen the general working relationships which in turn will promote better results.

Stress Management Techniques:

In the relentless hustle and bustle of the professional world, external stressors often act as catalysts for self-sabotaging behaviors. To navigate this tumultuous terrain, the mastery of stress management techniques becomes a vital skill. Consider these strategies as part of your toolkit for cultivating resilience in the face of these external pressures:

- **Me time:** Start by trying to include what I like to call 'Me time' into your schedule. If you are in charge of your work time and it's planning include at least one thirty-minute of 'Me time' into your working day. Planned time to dedicate to yourself is not a selfish act. By focusing on yourself, you can decide which activity you need to undertake to make your day more positive and productive. You can also use this time for self-development, training, or research. It's your time, make it flexible, and don't ever squander it.

- **Mindfulness Practices:** Embed mindfulness practices into your daily routine to anchor yourself in the present moment. Mindfulness techniques, such as meditation or mindful breathing exercises, act as a pause button amid the whirlwind of chaos. They offer a sanctuary of calm, allowing you to observe external stressors without immediately reacting.

- **Deep Breathing Exercises:** The simple act of deep breathing can be a powerful antidote to stress. Incorporate deep breathing exercises into your routine, especially during high-pressure situations. This intentional focus on breath not only oxygenates your body but also calms the nervous system, promoting a more composed response to external triggers.

- **Regular Breaks:** In pursuing professional excellence, the notion of taking breaks might seem counterintuitive. However, regular breaks are essential for recharging your mental and emotional faculties.

Use breaks to engage in activities that bring joy or relaxation, whether it's a brief walk, listening to music, or practicing a hobby. These interludes act as pressure valves, releasing accumulated stress and preventing it from morphing into self-sabotage. Take these moments to also make sure that you stay hydrated as this will help balance your body's physical needs as well as your emotional ones.

Boundary Setting:

The delineation between work and personal life is crucial for preventing external stressors from infiltrating your inner sanctum. Establishing clear boundaries is akin to creating a protective shield that safeguards your personal space and well-being. Consider these approaches to fortify the boundaries:

- **Defined Work Hours:** Set defined work hours and adhere to them diligently. When the workday concludes, consciously disengage from professional responsibilities. This temporal boundary communicates a clear endpoint to work-related stressors, allowing you to transition into your personal life with greater ease. Work-life balance is a crucial step to improving not only your time outside work but also your time within it. You will be a far more balanced person equipping yourself with the inner fortitude to make better more reflective decisions. Remember you do not 'live to work', you 'work to live'.

- **Digital Detox:** In an era of constant connectivity, adopting periodic digital detoxes is paramount. Designate specific timeframes, perhaps evenings or weekends, for disconnecting from work-related communication channels. This intentional break from digital engagement provides a respite, reducing the permeation of work stressors into your personal life.

- **Leisure Activities:** Actively engage in leisure activities that signify the demarcation between work and personal time. Whether it's pursuing a hobby, spending quality time with loved ones, or immersing yourself in recreational pursuits, these activities reinforce the separation of spheres. They become anchors of joy and relaxation, counterbalancing the impact of external stressors such as work.

By integrating stress management techniques and setting firm boundaries, you construct a robust defense against the encroachment of triggers. These coping mechanisms not only shield you from the adverse effects of stress but also empower you to navigate professional challenges with resilience and grace.

Balancing Work-Life Harmony and Self-Care:

As we have stated achieving a moderated work-life balance is important to establishing a more centered life. Let's elaborate on that a little more. Self-sabotaging often occurs when we are at our most stressed or tired or possibly both. Our barriers to this nasty little devil are at their weakest when we are not operating at our peak, so getting the balance right is a key achievement to help reduce the opportunity for self-sabotage to sneak up on us. Here are some considerations on how to achieve that.

Chapter 11: Conquering Addictive Behaviors

"I have absolutely no pleasure in the stimulants in which I sometimes so madly indulge. It has not been in the pursuit of pleasure that I have periled life and reputation and reason. It has been the desperate attempt to escape from torturing memories, from a sense of insupportable loneliness and a dread of some strange impending doom." [1]

Addictive Behaviors and Self-Sabotage

---

1. Edgar Allan Poe, 1842, The Masque of the Red Death

In the intricate landscape of personal growth, the bat-tleground marked by addictive behaviors and unbridled emotional responses can be a formidable challenge. This chapter serves as a supporter, guiding you through the exploration of addiction roots, unruly anger triggers, and, most importantly of all, strategies to conquer these adver-saries for all time.

Understanding the Roots of Addiction and Anger Triggers:

Before we embark on the journey of conquering addictive behaviors and mastering emotional regulation, it's impera-tive to unmask the elusive triggers that set these challenges into motion. Just as with other self-sabotaging tendencies, triggers can be the whispering voices from our past, un-resolved traumas, or coping mechanisms that have gone awry. Through self-reflection and a deep dive into our emo-tional landscape, these triggers can be revealed. This act lays the groundwork for future targeted interventions.

Navigating the Maze of Addiction:

Addiction, whether it's to substances, behaviors, or thought patterns, often finds its roots in a complex inter-play of genetic, environmental, and psychological factors. Understanding this intricate web is the first step towards dismantling it. It's not merely about breaking free from the chains of addiction but also about addressing the voids that these behaviors sought to fill. One is the symptom, the other the cause. By acknowledging this multifaceted nature of addiction, we pave the way for a more holistic recovery.

Here I will not repeat the R for Reflect as it is intentionally identical for all symptoms of self-destructive behavior. The key here is to delve deep within yourself to understand not just the triggers but also the behavioral drivers.

Take your time and use the exercises from earlier to seek this deep level of understanding. This form of self-destructive behavior can be deep-seated and hard to get to grips with. Moreover, it is also an area where we often find it hardest to accept. If this is the form that your self-sabotaging takes then start by asking yourself why you have decided to read this book in the first place. What outcomes made you seek it out? What were those negative outcomes related to? and what would you have changed in yourself, your behavior, or your reactions to avoid them? Where, when, and how many times before has your behavior caused such negative outcomes? Just by rationally going through each of these questions you will start to uncover the severity and long-term impacts.

Remember you are not alone. There are likely a good number of people that you know or have known who have suffered from self-sabotage. Many are probably still suffering. The BIG difference here is that you are doing something about it.

Just as you are not alone you can also seek others guidance and support in your journey. Some may have successfully navigated similar addictions such as substance abuse, drugs or alcohol, physical behavior, or emotional trauma. Seeking support is a strength to nurture, allowing awareness and acceptance to morph into the adoption of resolution strategies

Anger Management as Emotional Alchemy

Anger, the fiery emotion that courses through our veins like an unleashed volcano, is a formidable force, and yet, like a volcano much of its power is concealed beneath the surface waiting for the trigger to set it free upon the world. Addressing anger as a symptom and a potential catalyst for addictive behaviors necessitates a delicate approach to the complexities of human emotion. Instead of treating anger as a fearsome adversary to be fought and suppressed, we must embark on a transformative journey akin to emotional alchemy—turning the base metal of unbridled fury into the gold of constructive energy.

Understanding the roots of anger is sometimes complicated. It lurks deep within among unspoken emotions and unresolved conflicts. Anger, in its rawest form, is a signal—a red flag raised by our psyche, indicating that something is amiss, unaddressed, or wounded within us. It's a siren call for attention to the deeper layers of our emotional landscape. Therefore, the first step in this alchemical process involves peeling back the layers of anger to reveal the vulnerable core beneath.

Cultivating awareness around anger triggers requires introspection and an honest examination of the emotions that underlie its explosive mountain top. What lies beneath anger's surface may be fear, hurt, betrayal, or a myriad of other emotions that, when left unexplored, morph into the destructive force of rage. Unraveling these complex emotions is an act of self-discovery, requiring patience, compassion, and a willingness to confront our discomfort.

Think of the times that you have exploded with anger. How many of them were due to other people and how many were due to how you 'felt' inside about a certain event, behavior, or spoken word? What was really driving your extreme reactions? Was it more to do with you than with the other person? Was it how you had been feeling for a while waiting for a moment to gush forth like puss from an infected wound? If we are being truthful with ourselves we know that all that bad feeling was already within us. We were carrying it around just waiting for someone to expose it and set it free.

Once these underlying emotions are brought into the light, the alchemical process can begin, offering a transformative journey from the raw power of anger to more positive and constructive energy. Picture a canvas waiting to be painted or a blank sheet of paper eager to be filled with creativity. Creative expression can serve as a powerful outlet for the intensity of anger. Take, for instance, the frustrated soul who channels their anger into a vibrant piece of artwork, using colors and strokes to convey the depth of their emotions. The canvas becomes a testament to their inner struggles and, at the same time, a beautiful creation born from the ashes of anger.

Physical activities provide another avenue for this emotional alchemy. Consider the athlete who, in the crucible of a challenging workout, transforms the energy of their rage into drive, determination, and resilience. The rhythmic pounding of feet on the pavement or the focused effort in the weight room becomes a physical manifestation of their emotional release, a process of reshaping anger into strength and vitality.

Constructive communication becomes the spoken art in this transformative journey. Engaging in conversations that address the root causes of anger is akin to the sculptor carefully chiseling away excess material to reveal the refined form within. Picture two individuals sharing their vulnerabilities, expressing their feelings, and seeking understanding. Through dialogue, they navigate the intricate details of their emotions, reshaping the narrative from conflict to connection.

Imagine a couple in therapy, where they use communication as their meeting point to change their emotional drivers. Each session becomes a space for understanding, mutual empathy, and relationship growth. They address the underlying emotions that fuel their anger, molding their communication style into a constructive force that fosters intimacy and a deeper connection.

In the workplace, consider a team meeting where colleagues engage in open and honest discussions about the sources of their frustrations. Through constructive communication, they transform workplace tensions into collaborative solution-finding, reshaping the dynamics for a more positive and productive environment. They seek solutions and positive movement instead of being held stationary by frustration and resentment.

In the hands of emotional alchemy, anger ceases to be an overwhelming destructive force. Like a sculptor molding clay or an artist painting on a canvas, you can mold your anger into actions that reflect inner truths and desires for positive change. The destructive potential of anger is transmuted into a powerful force for good—a catalyst for personal growth and ongoing transformation, leaving behind a trail of creativity, resilience, and strengthened connections in its wake.

Techniques and Methods for Overcoming Addictive Behaviors and Managing Emotions

The very nature of addictive behaviors is that we are anchored to them as if they form a lifeline in the sea of life. They are repeating destructive forces that we drift toward whenever we feel the need. Generally, that need is driven by a trigger or response to something that we see as negative including our behavior. This is a habit-forming spiral of descent into the darkness of negativity and the destructive power of our own making. Let's be real here, addictive behaviors start with us. They are of our own making at least from the very outset. We all have choices and we can all make poor decisions, especially in times of heightened stress. We need to take responsibility for our actions and by accepting that responsibility do something about it. We all have the strength residing inside of us even if that journey looks long and bleak. We all can seek the light and the positivity of the person that we want to be.

Whether that destructive addiction is substance abuse, anger, or physical or emotional trauma there is always a way to escape its grip. Below are some exercises that you can use to help your journey upward from darkness to light.

Mindful Intervention: Navigating the Storm with Presence

In the vast expanse of our emotional sea, where addictive behaviors and unbridled anger create great turbulence in our lives, mindfulness stands as an unwavering lighthouse. An anchor point above the tumult, a beacon of positivity shining its beam across the rocks that can destroy our safe journey of life.

Exercise: Mindful Anchoring

(5 minutes)

Picture a serene moment: you, standing on the deck of your awareness, facing the crashing waves of craving. In this exercise, let's call it "Mindful Anchoring," find a quiet space and focus on your breath. Find a comfortable seat. Ensure that your feet are flat on the floor and try to relax. Close your eyes and begin to intentionally breathe deeply. As each breath flows in and out, visualize yourself anchored to the present moment. Feel the waves of craving rise and fall, but let your anchor hold you steady. Cultivate a feeling of calmness where you can simply be. Where the stressors of the day just flow past and you feel at one with yourself removing the need for your craving. This practice fosters self-awareness, cultivating the resilience needed to navigate life's tempests.

Cognitive Restructuring: Reshaping the Narrative

Our thoughts shape our actions, and in the realm of addiction and emotional challenges, cognitive restructuring is the process used to reshape the narrative of our thoughts. Let's engage in the "Thought Gardening" exercise to learn how we can change the way we feel.

Exercise: Thought Gardening

(15 minutes)

Take a moment to jot down recurring negative thoughts related to your addictive behavior or anger triggers. Now, challenge the first thought by reframing it with a positive or neutral perspective. Once you have noted down a different perspective, go to the next thought and keep repeating until all of the original list of thoughts has been reshaped. Read back through the list trying to feel those new more positive thought expressions. It's like pulling out the weeds of negativity and planting the seeds of healthier thoughts. This exercise will help you dismantle the foundations of destructive behaviors, allowing a garden of positive emotions to bloom.

Emotional Regulation Toolkit: Instruments for Serenity

Crafting a personalized emotional regulation toolkit is an empowering journey, offering you instruments for navigating the stormy seas of your emotions. Let's dive into the "Sensory Symphony" exercise.

Exercise: Sensory Symphony

(5 minutes)

Identify three key positive items that appeal to your senses —sight, touch, and smell. These could be for instance a comforting picture of happiness, a soft piece of fabric, or a calming scent each related to moments of joy and comfort. Keep these items in your emotional toolkit. In moments of heightened emotions, take a moment to engage with each item deliberately. Study the picture, touch the fabric, and smell the alluring scent. This sensory grounding helps you to navigate turbulent feelings, providing a pathway to serenity. Your toolkit becomes a source of comfort, a companion for the journey through emotional turbulence, and a counterbalance to any cravings.

These exercises, woven into the fabric of the R.E.L.E.A.S.E. process, offer innovative tools for you to not just understand but actively engage in your journey toward conquering addictive behaviors and mastering emotional regulation. Each exercise is a bright light, guiding you through the intricacies of your emotions, fostering growth, and illuminating the path to a more fulfilling and empowered life.

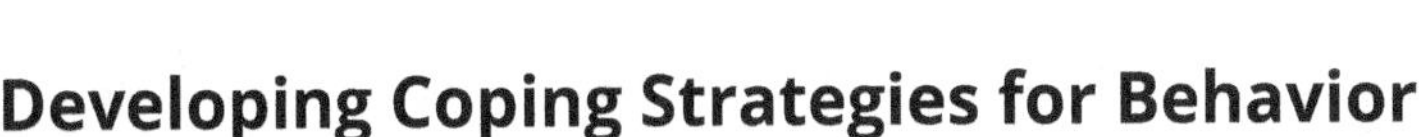

Developing Coping Strategies for Behavior Management

Navigating the Emotional Boxing Ring: Craftsmanship in Self-Regulation

Emotional self-regulation mirrors the craft of a seasoned boxer, dodging, weaving, and strategically engaging with emotions in the metaphorical boxing ring. It's not about suppressing your emotions but developing a keen awareness and crafting effective counter-moves to maintain balance in your life.

Exercise: Emotional Boxing

(5 minutes)

In this detailed exercise, "Emotional Boxing," identify three emotions linked to your addictive behaviors or anger triggers. Picture each emotion as an opponent in the ring. Now, devise specific counter-moves for each emotional 'opponent.' For example, if frustration surfaces, your counter-move might be a deep breathing technique. If anger begins to well up perhaps taking time to sidestep and walk away from your opponent to reposition for your next move would be a good counter. Practice these techniques regularly to enhance your emotional agility and responsiveness. Note down how they work in moments of stress or when you feel your trigger being pulled. Practice them allowing them to become habit-forming.

Personal Chronicles: Forging Your Testimonial Saga

Real-world testimonials are not just stories; they are chronicles of resilience and triumph.

Exercise: Chronicle Forming

(60 minutes)

In the "Chronicle Forging" exercise, become the author of your own testimonial saga. Reflect on significant moments where you overcame addictive behaviors or effectively managed your anger. Write a comprehensive narrative for each, delving into the emotional landscape, the challenges faced, and the ultimate victories gained. This exercise is a profound exploration of your journey, showcasing your achievements. Share this chronicle with your support network, transforming it into a source of inspiration for others facing similar challenges. Your narrative will become a force for good and a beacon of hope and shared strength.

These exercises, integrated into the RELEASE framework, empower you to not only comprehend but actively engage in the process of conquering addictive behaviors and mastering emotional regulation.

Conclusion

The battle with addictive behavior is a tough one. It can last all ten rounds but at the end of the bout if you can remain standing undaunted by situations that would have in the past triggered your negative emotional responses, then you are your own champion. Irrespective of the particular addiction it's the underlying root cause that needs addressing. The addiction itself is merely the outward symptom. Cure the root cause then the symptoms disappear.

Chapter 12: Ending Self-Sabotage

"It's not the situation that's causing your stress; it's your thoughts, and you can change that right here and now." [1]

Earlier in the book I mentioned the huge benefit of understanding the moments leading to self-sabotage. Not only the situations and the triggers but those early warning signs of rising emotions that act as precursors for self-sabotaging. Over the last days and weeks, you have spent a lot of time on introspection, reflection, understanding root causes, and the impact of self-destructive behavior when it occurs. You have also established coping mechanisms and ways to control self-sabotaging and have most recently read examples showing these strategies and methods in

---

1.

action. But what if you could anticipate self-sabotage before it even happened and preempt the situation altogether? How valuable would it be to stop self-sabotaging from happening at all?

Now that would be liberating, right?

Not only would you be armed with all the understanding of why you react in the way that you do, and what to do when those situations occur but you would be able to use that knowledge before those situations even arose. It's like 'Back to the Future' without the bad hair days.

Let's take a look at this time-bending possibility.

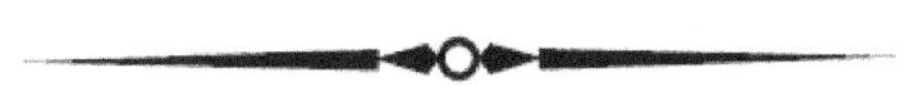

Telling the Tell

If you remember back in Chapter Seven you undertook some exercises that identified the situations, triggers, and emotions that you encountered when and just before self-sabotaging jumped up to ruin the day. We also discussed those feelings experienced as you started reacting to the situation you found yourself in. These could be; nervousness, blood rushing to your head, getting hot and feeling bothered, or simply a rising level of anger. This is your 'Tell'. The moment when a self-sabotaging event is about to strike. Each person's response will be different from others and potentially for different situations, we are after all wonderfully unique. However, if we use that knowledge of our tell to our advantage we can effectively preempt self-sabotage and rewrite our future.

Think about all those past situations when you have succumbed to self-sabotage and have made a decision that you later look back on and thought, "I wish I hadn't said that", or, "I wish I hadn't reacted in that way", or simply, "Shit!". How many opportunities would you have had to change your future? How many arguments or misunderstandings could you have avoided if you had only changed your approach or not reacted to certain remarks or situations? Generally, when we reflect on those events or situations we attempt to rationalize them or shift the blame but deep down we know that we could have done better. We could have been better.

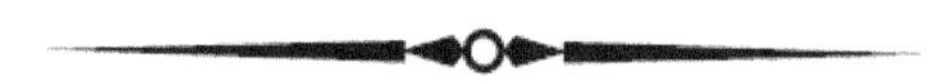

Gaining Your Super-Power

So how can you effectively bend time and assert your defensive measures against your self-sabotage before the situation occurs? That my friends is a very good question. And guess what I have the answer. The skill relies upon you recognizing your 'tell' for any given situation where you may react negatively and destructively.

Start by attuning your mind to feeling those moments as they materialize. The moment when a discussion with your partner starts to diverge into a disagreement, the times when you're in a meeting and you start to feel the first prickles of anger, the point where your heartbeat quickens when confronting a neighbor, or when your thoughts shift to addictive substances. These are all tale-tale signs that you need to tune into. Over the following weeks capture as many of those 'lead-up' moments and sensations as possible. Add these to your collected accounts until you feel that you have exhausted all the places, situations, encounters, conversations, and behaviors that act as precursors. Reflect on the list, memorize the learnings, and hold those learnings close because these will be your super senses ready to shout 'Now!" at a moment's notice when the next self-sabotage event is looming.

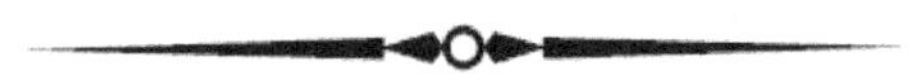

Changing your Future

You now have everything you need to bend time and change outcomes.

Here is a scenario that demonstrates this super-power in action:

Your partner gets in from work late. It's not the first time. They have been telling you that they are under pressure to deliver a piece of work which is really stretching them thin. However, you have been getting more and more agitated as it has occurred more frequently. You have never felt truly worthy of a great relationship and your lack of self-esteem only enhances your fears of your relationship failing. You may have been together for some time but could your partner be seeing someone else? You have already questioned them and they denied it as they had in the past when you last felt insecure, but those same insecurities are shouting from inside your head telling you that they are lying, that they are up to something, that this many late nights can only mean one thing. Tonight they are later than ever and you rush to meet them at the door not to welcome them home after a long exhausting day but to flat out accuse them of what you suspect. You can feel the anger rising along with the fear that everything is about to collapse around you. Your blood is pumping hard, you feel hot and you know what will shortly happen. You recognize the warning signs of self-sabotage and it's about to strike.

This is the point that your super senses kick in. This is the moment of inflection.

Based on previous experience you will launch into an angry confrontation and accusation which will spiral out of control on a wave of hysteria and ferocious fury. Things will be said that can never be retracted and the relationship will probably not survive. This is the immediate future expectation.

But wait, hang on just a split second because you have just learned all about your self-sabotage and the fact that it feeds off of fear, anger, and self-loathing. Suspicion and accusation are where self-sabotage loves to hang out waiting to ruin a life. You know all about this because you have just finished reading a great book on the subject by me and you are prepared. Your super sense leads seamlessly to your superpower. You have already rehearsed your coping mechanisms for such an occurrence. You breathe deeply and decide that your fighting move is to dodge to the left and reposition yourself in the ring of battle which in this instance means you stay put in the living room and wait for your partner to join you. Meanwhile, because you are taking the chance to breathe deeply and think about things you realize that self-sabotage is using your deep-seated root causes against you. He knows that you fear loss and rejection just as much as you feel undeserving of a loving relationship. But that was the past. You have spent time coming to terms with those feelings and the root causes of being abandoned as a child. You know self-sabotage wants to make you lonely and afraid and repeat the habit-forming behavior that has broken every relationship that you have ever had. You are aware of its intentions and what it has done to you in the past and you have accepted the challenge to not let it do it again. The actions you have adopted are there to vanquish self-sabotage before it can even start.

Now because your brain is an amazing piece of biological engineering that works faster than a speeding helicopter you would have completed this thought process in less time than it took to remain seated on the sofa. This allowed your partner to come in and calmly explain why they were late. Through open dialogue, you confide in them your fears and your deep-seated root causes. Through this truly intimate conversation, you realize that your partner is equally as desperate to ensure that their work does not encroach on your relationship and will do everything possible to make you feel safe and secure in a loving and faithful relationship.

Conclusion

Through using the R.E.L.E.A.S.E. Framework and by following the transformation process of awareness through to adoption you have managed to acquire the skills needed to confront and overcome your self-sabotaging tendencies before they can even start. The best news is that by achieving this you are creating positive habit-forming beliefs. Through regular repetition, you will be reaffirming the power of your new approach forming a virtuous circle of positivity that will thwart any reoccurrence of self-sabotage in the future.

Congratulations!

But the story isn't over there. To ensure that this is a sustainable process we need to cultivate the right environment and support mechanisms to keep you positive and in charge of your emotions as well as your behavior. Not only that but we need to explore the last parts of the two systems that we are following, Advocate and Empower.

I will see you in the next exciting chapter.

Now go and practice your new-found superpower.

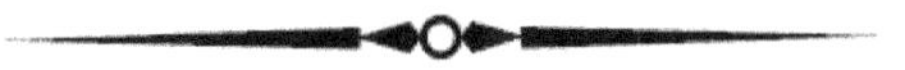

Chapter 13: Cultivating Self-Compassion and Personal Growth

"As a tree grows from its roots, so does personal growth flourish when rooted in the soil of self-compassion." [1]

In the world of personal evolution, cultivating self-compassion and fostering continuous personal growth are the key components that form resilience, strength, and fulfillment

---

1. Jackson James, (2024) End Self-Sabotage and Stop Fighting with Yourself!

within our lives. This chapter embarks on a journey to unravel the techniques and strategies that will empower you to nurture self-worth, embrace self-compassion, and bid farewell to the lingering specter of self-criticism.

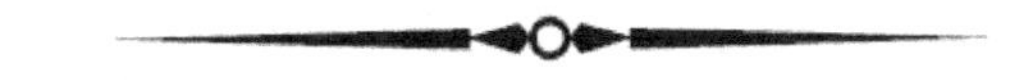

Fostering Self-Compassion and Self-Worth

As we move into the final E of Empower in the R.E.L.E.A.S.E. framework it's worth taking a moment to pause and examine just how far you have traveled.

The goal was to control your self-sabotaging tendencies, but to do that you first needed to reframe the whole issue, treating those tendencies as unwelcome symptoms to a more powerful underlying root cause. A bit like bad breath and tooth decay when the problem is that we simply don't like brushing our teeth. However, before you could achieve that you needed to form an awareness of the issues that self-sabotaging had caused. This was achieved in Chapter 1, through introspective, reflective exercises. By delving into your past and re-examining the decisions made you gained the understanding needed to be aware of the problems caused and the acceptance that you needed to act differently to overcome them.

By focusing on the decision triggers you began to recognize the emotional drivers of negative behavior. By establishing the root causes of your emotions and the situations which triggered them you were able to reassess your behavior and establish ways to predict it. You explored techniques to fight the onset of self-sabotage and sought help also from your subconscious dream state. to rehearse responses for better outcomes.

Through the integration of the R.E.L.E.A.S.E. framework into your life, you were able to deal with past trauma and those emotional drivers to reshape your behavior. By letting go of the past and embracing the future you journeyed on to adopting practices for ending self-sabotage. You also examined three core scenarios where self-sabotage is most likely to impact, relationships, work environment, and addictive behavior, with each demonstrating the key activities needed to overcome them.

Congratulations you are effectively evolving your mindset to seek solutions and support whilst aligning your entire being to use them in the most effective ways possible. These actions are the expressway on-ramps to personal development and empowerment. But to reach our final destination we must first make a pitstop at a friendly services pull-in, avoiding the dodgy roadside diner and overpriced memorabilia to focus on ourselves and our self-compassion to help us stay the course.

Self-compassion is not a get-out-of-jail-free term nor is it a selfish act. Yes, we have done some bad things. Most of those things have ultimately been detrimental to ourselves as well as those around us. For that, we must repent, however, the act of forgiveness must first start far closer to home. It must start with forgiving ourselves and introducing self-compassion into our lives.

Here are some ideas on how you can do that.

Self-Compassionate Mirror Exercise:

- Stand in front of a mirror and look straight into your own eyes. Speak to yourself with kindness, acknowledging your strengths and areas for growth. This direct, compassionate self-talk can foster a positive self-image.

Values Clarification Activity:

- Create a list of your core values—the qualities and principles that are important to you. Reflect on how aligning your actions with these values can lead to purposeful growth. Consider the specific steps that you can take to embody these values in your daily life. Embrace the actions that you have already taken and congratulate yourself for being on the journey.

Photographic Reflections:

- Compile a collection of photographs that represent key moments in your life where personal growth occurred. Create a visual timeline and reflect on the positive lessons learned from each experience.

This exercise provides you with a tangible reminder of your resilience and the progress that you have made and continue to make.

Compassion-Focused Meditation:

- Practice a compassion-focused meditation where you intentionally cultivate feelings of warmth and kindness towards yourself. Imagine a compassionate figure or mentor offering words of support and encouragement. This meditation promotes self-compassion and emotional well-being.

Random Acts of Self-Kindness:

- Engage in random acts of self-kindness throughout your week. These can be simple gestures like taking a break to enjoy a cup of coffee, permitting yourself to rest, or engaging in a favorite hobby. These regular acts of self-kindness contribute to a nurturing environment for personal growth. I also link them to specific activities that I need to undertake so they also act as self-provided encouragement and reward.

These self-compassion exercises and others mentioned earlier can add much-needed balance to your life providing positivism to counter the darkness of negativity. These highlight the good aspects of your life which are often overshadowed by negative habit-forming thinking.

Realizing that not everything is negative is a great start to embracing a life without the need for self-sabotage.

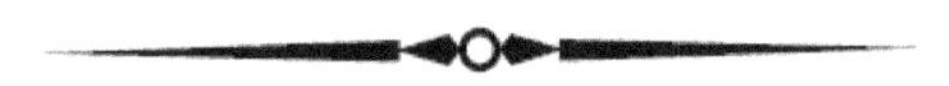

Continuous Personal Growth Strategies

So now you know how to incorporate self-compassion into your life but to carry that momentum forward you need to set personal growth strategies too. By creating growth goals that support you in becoming your future self, you will be addressing your behavior at the same time in manageable stages.

Growth goals:

Craft goals that align with your values and aspirations that you have already captured. Instead of succumbing to societal expectations, set objectives that resonate with your authentic self. Whether they involve professional achievements, personal milestones, relationships, or skill development, purpose-driven goals will aid continuous personal growth.

Lifelong Learning:

Embrace the philosophy of lifelong learning as a cornerstone for your growth strategy. Engage in diverse experiences, acquire new knowledge, and actively seek opportunities for intellectual and emotional expansion. The pursuit of learning not only broadens your perspectives but also fuels a sense of curiosity and accomplishment that propels you forward.

Resilience Building:

View challenges not as roadblocks but as stepping stones for personal growth. Cultivate resilience by reframing setbacks as opportunities for learning and adapting. Resilience is not the absence of difficulties but the ability to navigate them with grace and emerge far stronger on the other side.

Tools for Self-Improvement

Designing a toolkit with strategies and techniques to empower you in sculpting a life rich in self-worth and continuous improvement is a great motivator. These tools are not mere instruments; they are companions in the journey of self-compassion, offering practical strategies to elevate your well-being. The path to self-improvement is a dynamic one, uniquely shaped by your aspirations, challenges, and triumphs. Each tool presented here is a way to navigate the intricate steps of self-discovery and enhancement.

From immersive sensory exploration to intentional skill-building, these exercises provide a holistic approach to your personal growth. They encourage you to delve into the depths of your self-awareness, construct purposeful plans, seek mentorship from others, and engage in transformative reflection. Let these tools be your allies, crafting a narrative of self-improvement that resonates with authenticity and supports your continued evolution.

Personal Development Plans:

Develop a comprehensive personal development plan by breaking down your goals into specific, measurable, achievable, relevant, and time-bound (SMART) objectives. Identify short-term and long-term milestones, considering both the professional and personal aspects of them. Regularly revisit these plans and adjust them as you progress, ensuring their relevance to your evolving aspirations.

Mentorship and Support:

Take a proactive approach to seeking mentorship by identifying individuals whose journeys align with your goals. Consider mentors from diverse backgrounds to gain varied perspectives. Establish a mentorship agreement that outlines the expectations with regular check-ins, and areas of focus. Additionally, actively contribute to a supportive community, sharing your insights and learning from others' experiences.

Goal-Oriented Visualization Techniques:

Enhance your growth journey through goal-oriented visualization. Close your eyes and vividly visualize yourself achieving specific milestones. Engage your senses, emotions, and surroundings in your mental imagery. Regularly revisit these visualizations to reinforce your commitment to continuous progress.

Holistic Wellness Assessment:

Conduct a holistic wellness assessment covering various dimensions of well-being, including physical, emotional, social, intellectual, and spiritual aspects. Identify areas that require attention and create action plans for holistic self-improvement. Balancing these dimensions contributes to overall personal growth and fulfillment.

Feedback Strategies:

Actively seek and integrate feedback and support from diverse sources, including mentors, peers, and self-assessment. Constructive feedback provides you with valuable insights into areas for improvement and guides your personal development efforts. Develop a feedback integration strategy that involves regular feedback sessions and actionable steps to address identified areas.

Intentional Skill Building Activities:

Engage in intentional skill-building aligned with your personal development goals. Identify specific skills related to your professional and personal aspirations and immerse yourself in purposeful learning experiences. This hands-on approach accelerates your skill acquisition and reinforces a commitment to continuous improvement.

These tools will support your personal development creating a solid foundation for your life which will deminish the opportunity for self-sabotage to assert any influence. Embrace the richness of the journey, knowing that you are developing your skills and knowledge base in the image of your future self.

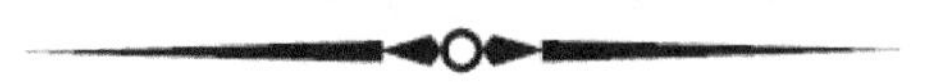

Chapter 14: Embracing Advocacy and Transformation

It's time to start living the life you've imagined[1]

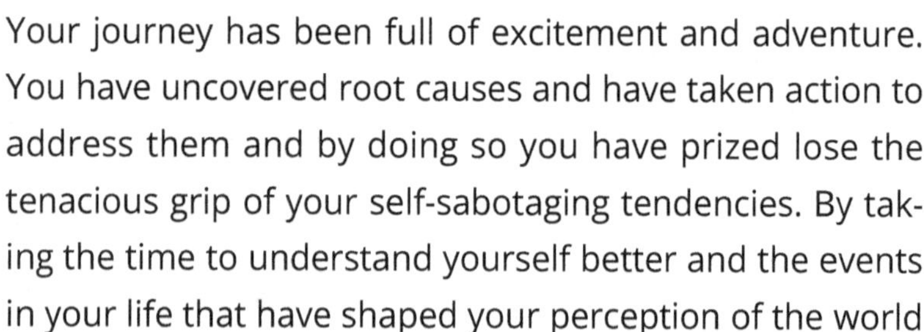

Your journey has been full of excitement and adventure. You have uncovered root causes and have taken action to address them and by doing so you have prized lose the tenacious grip of your self-sabotaging tendencies. By taking the time to understand yourself better and the events in your life that have shaped your perception of the world

---

1. Henry James (n.d.) As cited in James Jackson (2024) End Self-Sabotage and Stop Fighting with Yourself!

you have managed to overcome the emotive drivers and triggers that caused you to self-sabotage in the first place. By aligning your actions with your values and goals you have sought out your identified future self, imbued with all the attributes that you hold most dear. Along the journey, you may have gained help from trusted confidants or supporters who also held you accountable for the actions that you agreed. These steps have led to inner empowerment where you are equipped with all the right exercises and skills to forge new relationships, tackling self-sabotaging head-on wherever it may lurk.

I hope with all my heart that the preceding passage correctly describes your current state. If however, you have got to this point and still feel uneasy with the suggestions provided or your understanding of them, then I would ask you to go back to the start and reread each chapter slowly making copious notes. This is how I tend to do my topic research so guess what, you are not alone. Regroup around the fact that each observation or suggested exercise, is there for you to select from to create your unique solution. The descriptions should resonate with your soul but the exercises to exert control over your self-destructive tendencies are a personal and private thing. Pick the options that work with your personality, but also push your boundaries. Don't stay in your comfort zone which may feel all nice and cuddly but offers less development. Instigate things that you know will make you uncomfortable because you also recognize that growth needs change. You simply need the belief that you can be better and that you want to be that future self. So don't stop at merely reading about it, get out there and do it. Because transformation is truly in your gift. Grab it firmly by the hand and be reborn as the future self you want to be.

So after those rousing words, you may think that you are at the end of the book. You have after all covered the R.E.L.E.A.S.E. framework from acronym start to acronym end. Parallel to this we have also followed the change process from Awareness, through to Acceptance and then to Adoption but hey, wait a minute there is one more 'A' that we need to cover and that is the 'A' of Advocacy. I also associate the act of advocacy with sustainability, not the paper drinking straw type of sustainability, which may be good for the planet but terrible for sucking the last of your McDonald's shake through. No, the sustainability I'm referring to is the enduring kind that in this case means keeping to the program and ensuring that you never slip back into bad behaviors.

So with that introduction, I give you Chapter 14 Embracing Adocacy and Transformation, because transformational change is only ever good if it is sustainable change, forged with determination and commitment for the long term.

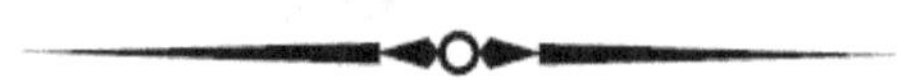

Commitment to Change and Self-Advocacy

Empowering the Architect Within

In the architectural blueprint of personal growth, commitment acts as the cornerstone. Imagine yourself as the architect, designing the structure of your transformation. Commit not just to change but to become the master builder of your destiny for the long term.

Exercise: Vision for the long-term

(Variable)

In this exercise, I want you to spend time considering which changes you have made or intend to make to become your future self where self-sabotage holds no sway. Form a personal commitment to these changes of behavior. in a visual form so that you can refer to it even during the roughest moments. Which form this visual representation takes is up to you. It could be a vision board for you arty types with images and words that solidify your commitment. It could also form a written pledge or even a symbolic object. Place it where you'll encounter it daily, a tangible reminder of your dedication to self-advocacy and continued transformation.

Exercise: The Pledge of Self-Advocacy

(10 minutes)

If you chose a different path in the last exercise then also craft a personal pledge—a manifesto of self-advocacy. This is your declaration to navigate the tides of self-sabotage with resilience and compassion. Consider it as a promise to stand up for your well-being and support others on their journeys. Now share this pledge with a trusted friend or confidant. This solidifies your commitment to the external world. This exercise not only reinforces your dedication but also invites accountability and shared support. It's harder to renege on something when someone else is holding your feet to the fire.

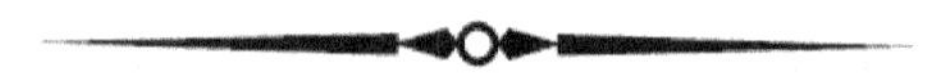

Empowerment through Self-Advocacy

The Mirror of Affirmations

Self-advocacy often begins with self-perception. If you tend to have a low self-perception then your determination for change may be fragile. To strengthen this I want you to relook at an earlier exercise as part of a daily ritual ideally first thing in the morning or just before you leave for work.

Exercise: Mirror of Affirmation:

(1 minute)

Each day spend a few moments in front of the mirror. This is not for last-minute grooming, this is for a far deeper level of awareness of yourself. As you intently study your face reflect on moments of triumph and success, reinforcing the narrative of your strength and determination. This isn't about reciting generic affirmations but acknowledging the unique qualities that make you resilient. Include any challenges that you have overcome in your drive to remove self-sabotage from your life. Know deep down that you are winning, improving, and moving forward irrespective of the prevailing winds of circumstance. You have the power to change your life.

This exercise fosters a positive self-image and strengthens the foundation of self-appreciation and self-advocacy.

Empathetic Listening Expedition

The empowerment that you are starting to experience extends beyond your being—it also encompasses those on parallel journeys. Practice empathetic listening by engaging in conversations with others facing similar challenges. Create a safe space where stories can be shared without judgment. This exercise not only offers support to others but also reinforces your role as an advocate whilst allowing you to understand a variety of viewpoints and experiences.

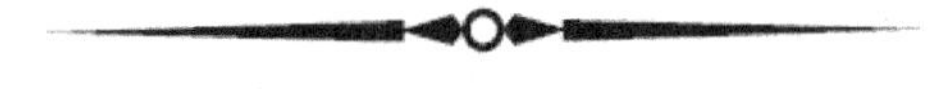

Advocacy Resources and Tools for Continued Support

Creating Advocacy Toolkits

To support your onward journey to a self-sabotaging-free future begin by equipping yourself with a personalized advocacy toolkit. This collection of resources, exercises, and insights gathered on your transformative journey could also include articles, books, and practical tools that you have found particularly empowering. This toolkit is not only a rich personal resource but a valuable asset to share with others. The act of curating this toolkit reinforces your commitment to your continued growth and advocacy of the journey that you have undertaken whilst also offering a tangible means of long-term support.

Virtual Support Networks

In this digital age, advocacy transcends physical boundaries. Explore virtual support networks—online communities, forums, or social media groups that are dedicated to personal growth and self-development. Engage with these by sharing your insights and learning with others. This exercise broadens your advocacy reach and provides continuous support and inspiration for those seeking to rid self-sabotage from their lives.

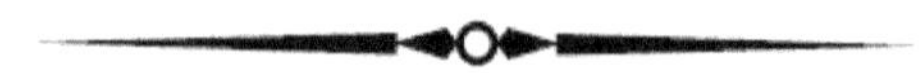

Conclusion:

The responsibility to maintain your commitment to controlling your self-destructive tendencies is yours to bear.

By using the suggested solutions you are shoring up your emotional resistance whilst embracing the change you feel inside. Sustainable change is your goal and by achieving that goal you can craft a life ready for greater success and happiness.

By advocating that change to others you will be playing your part in helping broaden this transformation. Help others and in so doing help yourself to maintain your long-term commitment.

Good luck on your journey to finding your future self and say a big "Hi" from me.

Jackson James

Chapter Fifteen

Chapter 14: Jackson's Awesome Extra Slice

"Happiness can be found even in the darkest of times if one only remembers to turn on the light."[1]

Surprise! Just when you thought it was all over...

1.

J.K. Rowling, (1999), "Harry Potter and the Prisoner of Azkaban"

Yep, I've got something more and very exciting for you all. I'm calling this **'Jackson's Awesome Extra Slice'** for no other reason than I think it sounds pretty cool and I've just had tea and cake. Yep, my fingers are worn down to mere stumps. Still, though, I have crafted some great additional content for you that I have been thinking about for a while. You may find its inclusion in future books, so you can be ahead of the curve and get your hands on it before anyone else and completely FREE from my publisher's website, 3eyepublishing.com, under the resources section. Or if you are reading this on your funky digital device you can click 'HERE' and read all about me (or skip that part) and go straight for the freebie section under resources where you can get your free 'Extra Slice'. I certainly hope that you enjoy it and you can always leave a comment or at least your details so that my publisher can feel all warm and cuddly inside that they have some subscribers and you will feel good because you will get to know when the next book launches. Win-win!

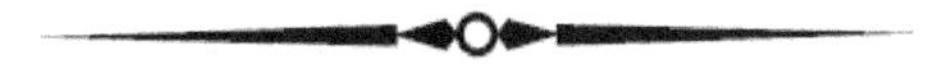

Book Reviews

Now this is where I need your help, or rather the other 8.1Bn residents on this fast-moving space ball do. We need to get the word out there that those who suffer from the onslaught of self-sabotage can rid themselves of the affliction by taking some of the hearty advice neatly cocooned in this small but friendly book. One way to do that is for each of you who have found this book either enthralling, entertaining, or perhaps enlightening to go out and purchase ten further copies and give them away to the first people you meet. Why? Well, because it is certainly likely that at least one of those receivers of such literary goodness will be suffering from the same thing as you were before you picked up a copy. This will not only help them but also help with your advocacy. Next, the nine who don't suffer from self-sabotage will almost certainly know at least one person each who could do with a helping hand on the subject and pass it on. This approach I would highly recommend.

Another way is to simply pop over to Amazon and provide an amazing book review so that when other seekers of self-sabotaging solutions start their search they will know that salvation is close at hand and that you are all pointing them toward a world where self-destructive tendencies have been forever eradicated. Whilst this is not as great as option one it will certainly help others too.

Oh, and do check out my other book titles in the 'Also by' section that follows next.

...it is now.

Also By

"The universe operates through dynamic exchange... giving and receiving are different aspects of the flow of energy in the universe. And in our willingness to give that which we seek, we keep the abundance of the universe circulating in our lives." [1]

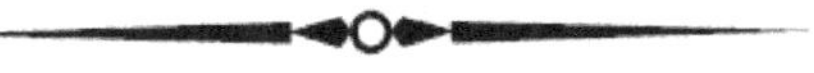

Hello Everyone!

Please find below details of my previous books which I think you would really like to get your hands on.

Buy your copy here: https://mybook.to/positivethinking

1.

The +Point: The Power of Positive Thinking for Everyone!

Ready for a life-changing journey filled with self-discovery, personal growth, and a positivity explosion that will blow your socks off?

If you suffer from any of the following then this book is for you:

1. **Stress**: Positive thinking helps manage stress by fostering a more optimistic outlook, reducing the impact of stressors, and enhancing resilience in challenging situations.

2. **Anxiety**: It will combat anxiety by promoting a more rational and balanced approach to handling worries and uncertainties, thereby reducing anxious thoughts and feelings.

3. **Depression**: Positive thinking will counter depressive thinking by shifting focus towards more hopeful and uplifting perspectives, aiding in managing depressive symptoms.

4. **Negative Self-talk**: It directly fights negative self-talk by promoting self-compassion, and self-acceptance, and encourages kinder more affirming

inner dialogue.

5. **Health Issues**: While it may not directly cure diseases, positive thinking supports better health outcomes by reducing stress-related physiological effects and bolstering your immune system.

6. **Low Self-esteem**: It combats low self-esteem by encouraging self-affirmation, recognizing your strengths, and fostering a more positive self-image.

7. **Fear and Uncertainty**: Positive thinking helps you to cope with fear and uncertainty by promoting a sense of resilience, adaptability, and a belief in your ability to overcome challenges.

8. **Relationship Conflicts**: It helps in managing relationship conflicts by fostering empathy, communication, and a more understanding attitude towards others, reducing conflict and tension.

9. **Procrastination**: Positive thinking combats procrastination by fostering a more motivated and goal-oriented mindset, leading to increased productivity and efficiency.

10. **Negative External Influences**: Positive thinking serves as a shield against negative external influences by allowing you to focus on the positive aspects of situations and resist being overly affected by negativity around you.

11. **Mild Fungal Foot Infection:** Thinking positively about fungal foot invasion may help take your mind off of it and come up with some alternatives to wearing Crocs.

More about the +Point Process

This revolutionary process has helped readers across the planet reshape their lives, transitioning negative thought processes to form repeatedly successful outcomes through proven positive thinking techniques and strategies.

This innovative process will help unearth your inner strengths, quell anxiety and stress, and discover your positive potential, empowering you to transcend existing limitations and attain unbridled success.

It will challenge existing beliefs, transform your outlook, and infuse your life with newfound purpose and vitality.

The +Point process will equip you with the right tools, strategies, and mindset needed to forge a brighter, more positive future, strengthening your emotional intelligence and driving your positive motivation.

Join the Positive Revolution sweeping across the planet!

Rethink your thinking, tap into boundless positivity, and embark on a journey like no other.

Buy your copy Here https://mybook.to/positivethinking

Scan Me to Buy Jackson's Great Book

To all of the people who ever thought paper straws were the way forward.

About the Author

"I love deadlines. I love the whooshing noise they make as they go by."[1]

Jackson James

Jackson James, is a maverick wordsmith, a citizen of the world who's navigated more continents than most people do in a game of Risk. Hailing from the bustling labyrinth of London, UK, and educated at Cambridge, Jackson the eternal student has devoted several lifetime's efforts to the pursuit of knowledge, culminating in a masterful under-standing of Psychology and Human Interaction. To keep things balanced he later added 'Positive Psychology' to his academic repertoire boosting his Scrabble word score by 37– *an act of sheer linguistic genius!*

---

1. Douglas Adams, 2002, "The Salmon of Doubt"

His eclectic career reads like an anthology of genres, from retail to tech wizardry, to consulting across global conglomerates. While others may puzzle over the complexities of modern gadgetry, Jackson chose to venture into the even more intricate terrain of human behavior and psychology. Recently taking the ultimate plunge, diving headfirst into the mysteries of unconventional thinking, dissecting the enigmatic human psyche, and sharing his findings through his writings.

His work is a multi-dimensional mirror reflecting the intricate tapestry of the human experience. Within its threads, you'll find elements of self-discovery, personal growth, and visionary leadership. But this isn't just about the mind; it's also about embracing the heart, the spirit, and a relentless passion for life's most profound mysteries.

Today, Jackson wears several jaunty hats – writer, life coach, mentor – and he wears them with the infectious enthusiasm of a true trailblazer. His unapologetically upbeat and quirky style is a magnet for those who dare to question the norm and explore the boundaries of their potential.

So, dear reader, embark on this journey with Jackson James and brace yourself for an expedition of enlightenment, hilarity, and unapologetic enthusiasm. Whether you're a seasoned explorer of the human psyche or a newcomer to the world of positive thinking.

JJ